*Research in
health promotion
and nursing*

Research in health promotion and nursing

Edited by
Jenifer Wilson-Barnett
and
Jill Macleod Clark

MACMILLAN

First published 1993 by
THE MACMILLAN PRESS LTD
Houndmills, Basingstoke, Hampshire RG21 6XS
and London
Companies and representatives
throughout the world

ISBN 0–333–60133–5 hardcover
ISBN 0–333–60134–3 paperback

A catalogue record for this book is available
from the British Library.

10   9   8   7   6   5   4   3
05   04   03   02   01   00   99   98   97   96

Printed and bound in Great Britain by
Antony Rowe Ltd, Chippenham, Wiltshire

Contents

Section Three: Developing the nurse's health promotion role

Section Four: The nurse's role in promoting healthy lifestyles

Section Five: Future directions

The contributors

Ms S.E. Adams
Service Manager
Bloomsbury and Islington Health
  Authority
Highgate Hill
London

Ms D. McCaffrey Boyle
Oncology Nurse Lecturer and
  Consultant
Washington, DC
USA

Mr M. Bradford
Research Assistant
Health and Social Policy Research Centre
Department of Community Studies
Brighton University of East Sussex
Lewes Road
Brighton
East Sussex

Mr C. Brooker
Regional Nurse, Research
Trent Regional Health Authority
Fulwood House
Old Fulwood Road
Sheffield

Mr J. Burden
Charing Cross Hospital
Fulham Palace Road
London

Professor A. Campbell
Professor of Biomedical Ethics
Biothics Research Centre
Otago Medical School
Dunedin
New Zealand

Dr A. Cribb
Lecturer in Education
Centre for Educational Studies
London

Ms A. Dines
Lecturer in Nursing Studies
King's College London
Strand
London

Ms K. Ferguson
Lecturer
Department of Nursing
Manchester University
Manchester

Ms M. Flatley
Research Student
Department of Nursing Studies
King's College London
Strand
London

Ms. J. Foulkes
Psychology Department
University of St Andrew's
Fife
Scotland

Ms U. Gallagher
Charing Cross Hospital
Fulham Palace Road
London

Ms J. Goodeve
Research Student
Department of Nursing Studies
King's College London
Strand
London

Professor J. Igoe
Associate Professor/Director
School Health Programmes
University of Colorado
Health Sciences Centre
Colorado
USA

Professor M. Johnston
Psychology Department
University of St Andrew's
Fife
Scotland

Ms K. Jones
Research Associate
Department of Nursing Studies
King's College London
Strand
London

Ms S. Kendall
Reader
Faculty of Health Studies
Buckinghamshire College
Queen Alexandra Road
High Wycombe
Bucks

Ms S. Latter
Lecturer
Department of Nursing Studies
Normanby College
King's College Hospital
London

Professor K. Luker
Department of Nursing
Liverpool University
Rodney House
70 Mount Pleasant
Liverpool

Mr J. Lunney
Nurse Science Administrator
Health Promotion/Disease
   Prevention Branch
National Center for Nursing Research
Bethesda, MD
USA

Professor J. Macleod Clark
Department of Nursing Studies
King's College London
Strand
London

Ms M. Malone
Health Visitor
Lewisham and North Southwark
   Health Authority

Ms Julienne Meyer
Lecturer
Department of Nursing Studies
King's College London
Strand
London

Dr L. Meerabeau
Head of School of Advanced Nursing
North East Surrey College of Technology
Nescot
Reigate Road
Ewell
Surrey

Ms Marjaana Pelkonen
Senior Lecturer
Department of Nursing
University of Kuopio
Finland

Ms A. Pursey
Department of Nursing
Liverpool University
PO Box 147
Liverpool

Ms M. Renfrew
Midwife Researcher/Director
National Perinatal Epidemiology Unit
Oxford

Ms C. Robertson
Psychology Department
University of St Andrew's
Fife
Scotland

Ms K. Rowe
Department of Nursing Studies
King's College London
Strand
London

Professor K. Tones
Health Education Unit
Leeds Metropolitan University
Leeds

Ms J. Walker
Clinical Psychologist
Reader in Nursing Studies
Department of Nursing, Health and
   Community Studies
Bournemouth University
Dorset

Professor J. Wilson-Barnett
Department of Nursing Studies
King's College London
Strand
London

Ms S. Winn
Lecturer in Social Policy
Health and Social Policy Research Centre
Department of Community Studies
Brighton University of East Sussex
Lewes Road
Brighton

Introduction

Jenifer Wilson-Barnett and Jill Macleod Clark

This book of readings explores the subject of health promotion and its relationship to nursing and reviews research in this area which demonstrates the nature, effectiveness and extent of health promotion in practice. Internationally famous experts in the field are included in the list of more than twenty contributors which spans all areas of nursing, midwifery, health visiting and health education. As such this is the first collection of its kind! Most of the chapters are based on papers given at a very successful international conference, especially selected because of their rigorous research base and depth of understanding.

Aimed at senior students, practitioners and teachers in nursing and allied health care fields, this book will help to clarify terms and explain how health promotion can be integrated into practice and evaluated. The variety of topics covered is wide and the presentation of the material provides easy access for readers. Sections are introduced with linking passages which offer synthesis and commentary.

All the chapters discuss the relationship between nursing and health promotion, accepting that this is an important component of the nursing role. In the first chapter, Keith Tones demonstrates how political and economic factors impinge on health at every level. Awareness of this is essential when attempting to counter the effects of deprivation and adverse political forces. This is followed by the first of five sections in which theoretical and ethical issues are explored and in some chapters the philosophy of health promotion and nursing is challenged.

The second section on health promotion in practice demonstrates how far nurses have been able to adapt in order to reflect the values and openness required. Chapters in this section indicate that a fundamental shift in the process of providing care is necessary. Because health promotion is an enabling, empowering strategy, staff need to alter their perspectives and behaviour. Few seem able to do this as yet, but models of good practice are starting to emerge.

Good models clearly need to be described and replicated and the third section of chapters provides some beneficial directions. Mental health is also targeted in two of the contributions and while this area of practice may be seen as distinct, it is clear that principles and strategies may be very appropriate for more general application. For instance, stress management and the need for families to understand the factors involved in promoting or restoring healthy living pertain across most specialities.

Section four explains how nurses can intervene to aid those who have health problems using an explicit philosophy of health promotion. This involves moving away from the traditional health education process, when information giving was predominant, to a more sophisticated interaction which assists individuals to recognise their own choices. Clearly this may involve challenges to what is established but is probably much more worthwhile with enduring beneficial effects.

In the last section on future directions readers will probably be impressed by the level of financial investment provided in the USA and the apparent contrast in Great Britain, where sparse attention is given to sustaining occupational health services.

More encouraging, though, is the clear vision in the concluding chapter for future practice where clients are treated as equals, where their own capacities are recognised and where professionals give support based on a careful discussion and respect for particular needs and circumstances.

It is hoped that this volume will stimulate readers to reflect on the potential for improving practice among the health care professions. Although much of the research exposes inadequacies, this may provide motivation and hopefully more understanding of what changes are needed and, of course, of the many future challenges for research.

1 The theory of health promotion: implications for nursing

Keith Tones

Health promotion: anatomy and ideology

Health promotion is an idea which has been adopted with some enthusiasm in recent time; like virtue, it is considered to be a good thing but also like virtue it is not especially easy to define. In fact not only has the term been open to several interpretations (Tones, 1985, 1986) but some of these may actually derive from different ideological positions. For instance, the definition of health promotion underpinning the recent emergence of health promotion 'clinics' as part of the development of general practice in the UK is actually at odds with the main thrust of the World Health Organisation's formulation of the concept. The approach adopted in this chapter, on the other hand, seeks to incorporate the WHO's ideological position. It will, in addition, suggest a structural analysis which places health education at the very heart of health promotion. Indeed, the structural analysis of health promotion can be encapsulated in the simple 'formula': *Health Promotion = Health Education × Healthy Public Policy*. The major function of health education within this formula is considered to be one of *empowerment*. And so, in considering the health promoting role of nurses, the key issue would seem to centre on the extent to which nurses, and the settings in which they work, can contribute to the empowerment of patients, clients and the community at large.

The ideology of health promotion

The central values of health promotion have been elaborated by the WHO in its 1984 formulation and forged into a series of political statements by 200 delegates from thirty-eight nations in the form of the Ottawa Charter (1986). These initiatives were in turn based on the principles of Primary Health Care developed at the Alma Ata Conference (1978). The ideological perspective and its associated

ethical and moral view of humanity may be summarised in the
following principles and statements of belief:

- Health should be viewed holistically and as a positive state; it is also
  an essential commodity necessary for achieving the ultimate goal of
  a socially and economically productive life.
- Health will not be achieved or illness prevented and controlled
  unless we tackle successfully the substantial inequalities which exist
  between nations and within nations and social groups.
- A healthy nation is not only one which has an equitable distribution
  of resources but one which also has an active, empowered
  community which is vigorously involved in creating the conditions
  necessary for healthy people.
- Health is too important to be left to medical practitioners; there must
  be a 'reorientation of health services'. It is important to recognise
  that a wide range of public and private services and institutions
  influence health for good or bad. Moreover, medical services
  frequently do not meet the needs of the public; they often treat
  people as passive recipients of care and are thus fundamentally
  depowering. The main task of health promotion is to enable not to
  coerce; we should be concerned with cooperation rather than with
  compliance.
- People's health is not just an individual responsibility; our health is
  to a large extent governed by the physical, social, cultural and
  economic environments in which we live and work. To cajole the
  individual to take responsibility for his or her own health while
  ignoring the social and environmental circumstances which conspire
  to make them ill is victim blaming; it is not only unethical, it is
  inefficient. At the centre of health promotion is 'healthy public
  policy'.

The pivotal role of 'healthy public policy' is shown in *Figure 1.1*, which
also identifies what the Ottawa Charter considers to be the key
requirements for avoiding unnecessary disease and the achievement of
a socially and economically productive life.

The structure of health promotion

Turning our attention now to the 'anatomy' of health promotion, it is
self-evident that there must be a structure to facilitate the transformation
of the rhetoric of health promotion into practice. This can be done by
extending the often quoted Health Field concept (Laframboise, 1973)
from description into action. In short, this 'common-sense' notion
asserts that there are four major influences on health and disease:
individual genetic endowment; the health/medical services; individual

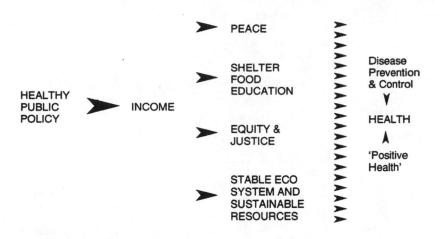

Figure 1.1 *Healthy public policy and the attainment of health*

behaviours or lifestyle; the physical, social, cultural and economic environment. Since the first of these is as yet not readily manipulated, health promotion must consist of the deliberate (and hopefully efficient) management of the other three 'inputs' to health. As we have noted, we would be wise to extend the definition of medical service so that it includes a wide range of services such as housing and transport. We should also work for the reorientation of these services so that they are user friendly; we should seek to demystify medicine as part of the process of demedicalisation and community empowerment. Again, to counter justifiable accusations of victim blaming, the focus of attention must shift from the individual to the environment and social structure. Our work with individuals should be one of enabling and supporting rather than cajoling and coercing; in short, the task is one of empowerment.

As was asserted earlier, the radical changes required by a true health promotion strategy must be paralleled by a change in policy — nationally and internationally, regionally, locally and at the level of organisations and institutions such as hospitals. Any 'radical shift in policy is notoriously difficult to achieve; perhaps the central tenet of the argument presented here is that it will not be achieved without effective health education operating at all levels.

The contribution of health education

The part played by health education has been more completely discussed elsewhere (Tones, 1987; Tones *et al.*, 1991). It is summarised in *Figure 1.2*.

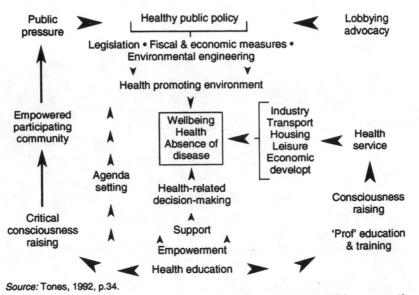

Source: Tones, 1992, p.34.

Figure 1.2 *The contribution of health education to health promotion*

In short, whereas the traditional functions of lobbying and advocacy (as described in the Ottawa Charter) may be used to bring about healthy public policy, their impact is inevitably limited by the prevailing power structure. For instance, at the time of writing, the UK government has successfully resisted the combined 'health' lobbies' efforts to have it support European Commission goals to ban all advertising and sponsorship of tobacco products. Accordingly, one of the most important tasks of health education is to create critical consciousness (Freire, 1970; Zacharakis-Jutz, 1988) and subsequently an empowered participating community which might exert powerful public pressure for change of policy – or, indeed, a change of government!

A second function of health education is indicated in *Figure 1.2* as 'professional education and training'. In addition to the well-established practice of providing health professionals with the skills and knowledge needed to communicate with and educate, for example, patients, the new health education task is (i) to convince a much wider range of occupational groups that they have a health promotion function (note earlier reference to housing and transport) and (ii) to press for a reorientation of health services.

The central strand of health education in *Figure 1.2* refers to traditional, individually focused health education. The emphasis of the 'new' health education is, however, not so much coercion and exhortation as facilitation and support. The assumption here is that we should remove those barriers which militate against free and healthy choices. Such an approach is consonant with those definitions of health promotion which declare that its major task is to 'make the healthy choice the easy choice'. Clearly it is the purpose of health policy to remove environmental and structural barriers to action. On the other hand, many barriers exist *within* the individual – including feelings of helplessness, low self-esteem, lack of skills and 'addictions' of one sort or another. The health education purpose here is one of self-empowerment – a notion which we will now seek to explore and define.

Empowerment and the concept of control

A full discussion of the relationship between empowerment and control is beyond the scope of this chapter and a more complete analysis is available elsewhere (Tones, 1992). No further reference will be made here to the notion of community empowerment and discussion will centre on the empowerment of the *individual* (*self-empowerment*). The dynamics of self-empowerment are complex but central to empowered action are the four following factors: (i) the environmental circumstances which may either facilitate the exercise of control or, conversely, present a barrier to free action, (ii) the extent to which individuals actually possess competences or skills which enables them to control some aspect of their lives and perhaps overcome environmental barriers, (iii) the extent to which individuals *believe* they are in control, and (iv) various emotional states or traits which typically accompany different beliefs about control – such as feelings of helplessness and depression or feelings of self worth. Let us first consider briefly the first of these four influences on self-empowerment – the influence of environment.

As indicated earlier, to ignore the importance of an adverse environment on health and illness is to be guilty of victim blaming. Much has been written about macro influences on health – such as poverty and other broader factors operating in society at large. For our present purpose we will focus more on the health promoting possibilities of an organisational milieu – such as the hospital. In this context one can do no better than refer back to Goffman's (1961) classic characterisation of the hospital as a 'total institution' with its tendency to depersonalise and disempower patients. More recently, Taylor (1979) noted that the hospital was one of the few places where an individual forfeits control over virtually every task he or she customarily performs. She then pointed out that patients adjust to this depowerment by adopting behaviours which causes staff to label them as either 'good patients' or 'bad patients'. Bad patients are those who demonstrate classic 'reactance' by rebelling against attempts to rob them of their control. Good patients, on the other hand, are those who approximate to Goffman's recommendation for the ideal patient role, namely, an inanimate state involving cheerful cooperation and dependency! Clearly, good patient behaviour – in so far as this represents a mode of adjusting to feelings of lack of control – is not healthy patient behaviour. On the other hand, it seems increasingly clear that believing that one has some kind of control over one's life is beneficial in many ways. Before we can identify strategies for empowerment, we need, however, to operationalise the concept of control and recognise some of the different dimensions in beliefs about control.

First, we should note that there is an important distinction between *believing* that we are in control and actually having the necessary power and competence to influence what happens to us. Lewis (1986) offered an interesting typology of control which is particularly relevant to the clinical context. She identified separately the following kinds of control: processual control, cognitive control, behavioural control, contingency control and existential control. The first of these describes the kind of situation in which, for instance, a patient might be 'consulted' about decisions but not actually have any real influence on that decision. Such tokenism may, however, be beneficial in that people like to *believe* they are exercising some degree of control even when the belief is illusory. Cognitive control has a clear psychological benefit: a patient who understands what is involved, say, in a painful investigative procedure may not actually be able to influence the level of discomfort but be in a position to manage the event intellectually and thus reduce its threatening properties. Behavioural control involves a patient actually acquiring some competence which provides some degree of real control over an event, for example, acquiring relaxation skills to reduce labour pains. The notion of contingency control is to all intents and purposes identical to Rotter's (1966) seminal notion of 'locus of control'. According to this notion, people vary in the extent to which they believe that what happens to them in life is due to either (i) their own efforts (internal locus of control) or (ii) the influence of chance and/or powerful others (external locus of control). Internality has been consistently associated with healthy behaviours or outcomes. A related but more useful notion is that of self-efficacy (Bandura, 1977): before patients who are recovering from a myocardial infarction commit themselves to a graduated exercise regime, they must actually believe they are capable of achieving the level of prescribed activity without experiencing a further heart attack.

The idea of 'existential control' is of special interest since it is in many ways different from the other kinds of control discussed so far. Indeed, it might be argued that it represents an acknowledgement of a lack of control: essentially it involves the imposition of meaning on (typically negative) occurrences. Even if patients do not believe they are in control of the illness or the treatment, the situation may be accepted with equanimity provided it can be explained in terms of some 'life philosophy' or set of religious beliefs. Accordingly, it may well be possible for people to believe that they lack control without suffering from the various negative health consequences, such as poor self-esteem and depression, which result from 'learned helplessness'. It would, however, be unwise to rely on this!

Health promotion and empowerment: some implications for nursing

In discussing the implications of the model of health promotion outlined here for nursing practice, two main issues will be raised. The first takes the form of an assertion that if nursing is to take health promotion seriously it must be actively concerned with the empowerment of clients and patients. The second issue is more problematic and takes the form of a question: to what extent can nurses legitimately be involved in political action to promote health? The latter question has a particular poignancy at the present time – at least in the UK – with recent discussions of the legitimacy of 'whistle-blowing' to draw attention to inadequacies in the provision of health care in the context of health services, where a concern with cost cutting may appear to have a higher priority than client welfare. Watts (1990) has argued unequivocally that the values underpinning nursing are synonymous with empowerment, community involvement and democratisation. The reality is that health promotion is fundamentally political and although it might not be a sensible career move for individuals to become political activists, professional bodies must surely lobby for healthy public policy in accordance with the principles of the Ottawa Charter. After all, Florence Nightingale established a sound precedent for critical consciousness raising.

As regards the empowerment of clients and patients, a full discussion of the role of nurses is not possible here. A few simple points may, however, be made about the requirements for a health promoting hospital. We should first, though, acknowledge that nurses working within the community are frequently involved in the work of health promotion and empowerment – typically through community development work. The focus here on the hospital is not meant to diminish the importance of the invaluable public health function of nurses outside the hospital but rather to emphasise the need for critical thinking on how health promotion might be implemented within the hospital setting.

We should first of all reiterate the importance of the complementary functions of policy and education. A hospital which seeks to promote health through empowerment must have a sound policy which might build on such notions as a Patients' Charter. However, it must go beyond bland statements about patients' rights and ensure that the hospital environment is conducive to empowerment – and that staff have the skills they need to educate for empowerment. Wuest and Stern (1991) described rather well the way in which parents of a group of children with otitis media became empowered carers. They moved from a state of 'acquiescing' and 'helpless floundering' to a point where they were confidently and efficiently managing their children's condition. Rather sadly this particular process of self-empowerment occurred in spite of the best efforts of the health professionals whose main contributions appear to have been to confuse and depower!

At the heart of the empowerment process is the twofold task of modifying patients' beliefs about control and providing them with whatever competences they might need to achieve this goal. It is gratifying to note evidence that empowerment strategies of this kind can be successful. For instance, in the context of acute care, a wealth of research on the provision of 'anticipatory guidance' prior to surgery or other stressful clinical procedures suggests that a number of desirable outcomes can be attained. These range from better mental health and reduced demand for analgesics to earlier discharge from hospital. While there is still uncertainty about the precise mechanisms involved, it seems clear that one or more of the various beliefs about control mentioned earlier appear to be central to the effectiveness of the interventions. Earlier discharge is clearly most desirable economically and should appeal to health services managers. While on this subject of cost effectiveness, it is worth noting in passing Taylor's (1979) encouraging observation that (in the USA) malpractice suits tend to be associated with patients' feelings of helplessness rather than their empowerment!

It will doubtless be self-evident that creating 'good' compliant patients is completely at odds with contemporary exhortations to take responsibility for your health and 'look after yourself'. It should be equally clear that the transfer of power to patients (and their carers) is a prerequisite for effective rehabilitation. For instance, appropriate self-efficacy beliefs about exercise are important in promoting recovery from heart attack (Ewart, 1992). And, more generally, the health of elderly people would also seem to be significantly related to notions of control and associated positive self-image (Reid *et al.*, 1977; Ryden, (1984). Indeed, the classic work of Langer and Rodin (1976, 1980) shows the two complementary processes of health promotion (policy and education) in action. Environmental modification and education designed to enhance control resulted not only in better quality of life of a group of institutionalised old people, but also seemed to improve their life expectancy.

One final point must be made. Any policy designed to achieve a health promoting hospital should be based on the notion of the hospital as a community of patients *and* staff. Its concern should, therefore, be to empower not only patients but staff too. There is nothing new in the suggestion that the nurse should act as a health promotion role model. It is quite common to advocate that nurses should set a good example by, for instance, not smoking. What is perhaps more novel is the idea that nurses should model empowerment. There are obvious implications in all that has been said so far about the health promotion role of nurses for training and the nurse curriculum. Not least is the suggestion that assertiveness training should form an important part of the repertoire of social and education skills which will support the nurses' health promotion function – and which will contribute to and reinforce the professional identity of the nursing profession.

References

Bandura, A. (1977). Self efficacy: toward a unifying theory of behavioral change. *Psychological Review, 84,* 2, 191–215.

Ewart, C. K. (1992). Role of physical self-efficacy in recovery from heart attack, in Schwarzer, R. (ed.). *Self-Efficacy: Thought Control of Action.* Hemisphere Publishing: Washington.

Freire, P. (1970). *Pedagogy of the Oppressed.* Continuum: New York.

Goffman, E. (1961). *Asylums.* Doubleday: New York.

Laframboise, H. (1973). Health policy: breaking the problem down into more manageable segments. *Canadian Medical Association Journal, 108,* 388–91.

Langer, E. J. and Rodin, J. (1976). The effects of enhanced personal responsibility for the aged. *Journal of Personality and Social Psychology, 34,* 2, 191–8.

Langer, E. J. and Rodin, J. (1980). Ageing labels: the decline of control and the fall of self esteem. *Journal of Social Issues, 36,* 2, 19–29.

Lewis, F. M. (1986). The concept of control: a typology and health related variables (unpublished MS scheduled for publication).

Reid, D. W., Haas, G. and Hawkings, M. E. S. (1977). Locus of desired control and positive self-concept of the elderly. *Journal of Gerontology, 32,* 4, 441–50.

Rotter, J. B. (1966). Generalized expectancies for internal versus external control of reinforcement. *Psychological Monographs, 80,* 1, 1–28.

Ryden, M. B. (1984). Morale and perceived control in institutionalized elderly. *Nursing Research, 33,* 3, 130–7.

Taylor, S. E. (1979). Hospital patient behavior: reactance, helplessness, or control? *Journal of Social Issues, 35,* 1, 156–84.

Tones, B. K. (1985). Health promotion – a new panacea? *Journal of the Institute of Health Education, 23,* 1, 16–22.

Tones, B. K. (1986). Health education and the ideology of health promotion: a review of alternative strategies. *Health Education Research, 1,* 1, 3–12.

Tones, B. K. (1987). Promoting health: the contribution of education, in *Education for Health in Europe.* Scottish Health Education Group: Edinburgh.

Tones, B. K., Tilford, S. and Robinson, Y. (1991). *Health Education: Effectiveness and Efficiency*. Chapman & Hall: London.

Tones, B. K. (1992). Health promotion, empowerment and the concept of control, in *Health Education: Politics and Practice*. Deakin University Press: Geelong, Victoria, Australia.

Watts, R. J. (1990). Democratization of health care: challenge for nursing. *Advanced Nursing Science, 12, 2*, 37–46.

WHO (1978). *Primary Health Care*. World Health Organization: Geneva.

WHO (1986). *Ottawa Charter for Health Promotion*. World Health Organisation: Geneva.

Wuest, J. and Stern, P. N. (1991). Empowerment in primary health care: the challenge for nurses. *Qualitative Health Research, 1, 1*, 80–99.

Zacharakis-Jutz, J. (1988). Post-Freirean adult education: a question of empowerment and power. *Adult Education Quarterly, 39*, 41–7.

SECTION ONE
Theoretical Issues

This first major section offers analysis of the concept of health promotion and a philosophical debate on the meaning and compatibility of health care and health promotion. Some contributions may seem contentious and difficult to contemplate, others challenge the reader to consider the conflict inherent within a system which respects autonomy and the aim of promoting a healthy community.

From a more general perspective which is also provocative Campbell poses quite fundamental questions, as do Burden and Gallagher. Equally challenging is the more specific scenario painted by Dines, which encourages the reader to take a position and analyse the consequences for practice and for their own personal integrity.

In essence this section confronts several issues on the limits or extent to which health promotion supports or negates free will. Intentionally, authors question established views, examine inherent contradictions in value systems and explore whether professionalism can be exploited positively and whether individual practitioners are cognisant of their own motivations and values.

2 The meaning of health promotion: a personal view

Jenifer Wilson-Barnett

Far more consensus on what 'health promotion' means has emerged over the last two years. This broad term refers to an approach and philosophy of care which reflects awareness of the multiplicity of factors which affect health and which encourages everyone to value independence and individual choice. Such a philosophy would also reject inequality in provision of resources to combat ill health and the imposition of one set of values, however, beneficent, upon another. Free will and the ability of individuals or groups of people to determine the way they live are therefore of supreme importance. The reassertion of such values within the context of health in the quality of life has become necessary to combat certain developments and health care provision and to publicise the growing evidence that inequality in socio-economic status is associated with variations in levels of health.

Meanings of terms such as 'health' and 'empowerment' need to be understood by health carers in order that their practice can reflect what is deemed to be positive. Living life in a way which is satisfying, fulfilling and helpful to others is probably important to us all. Maximising individual potential to enjoy the rich and varied opportunities that are available from social contact to many physical and intellectual pursuits is a shared goal in most cultures. Enabling people to aim for this should be the goal of many agencies but health professionals may be in a special situation to influence this.

For many who are at risk of deprivation, whether economic or personal, the support and resources available in the health services could be invaluable. In the past these have mainly been distributed in a way which reflected the priority of acute care. Even in the least developed and poorer countries acute medicine and hospital-based provision has tended to absorb the majority of the health budget. It is now becoming much clearer that far more fundamental investment in education and agriculture can reach a wider community and prevent epidemics of fatal disease. However, recent civil war in Somalia and Yugoslavia also serves to demonstrate that political stability and power can destroy the health of total populations.

By attempting to influence the positive value of good heatlh, happiness and self-determination, this philosophy of health promotion encompasses many activities and quite explicitly aims to inform as many as possible or 'spread the word' on how this may be effected. From public policy to individualistic care, specific principles should be established in order to guide practice. These involve a radical shift in the way care is provided and thereby require re-education of all involved. Breaking unhealthy habits of all kinds is necessary both by individuals who are engaging in risky behaviours and also by staff who are providing care which is not 'health promoting', because they are imposing their will and not respecting the choices of others.

Such principles or values need to be identified and this book aims to explicate them and demonstrate how they can be applied in the real world. Valuing independence, free will and choice accompanied by the provision of clear, useful and truthful information may sound familiar. However, such principles are not always omnipresent in health services. The inequalities within the system affect a culture where those in powerful positions can provide what they believe to be necessary, but this becomes established practice and may not reflect changing situations or priorities within a community. In a sophisticated and specialised system it is a huge challenge to redress the balance so that real choices are offered and those providing this choice genuinely believe that the recipients have the right to reject their advice.

Equality and democracy have been publicly upheld in Western societies for many centuries but their translation and implementation is often obscured or distorted. Political systems may have been constructed with checks and balances but these need to function on a daily basis throughout society. It is quite salutary to see the lack of democracy in many enterprises, as strict hierarchies exist in most large organisations. Preservation of individuals' rights against those in power is fundamental to justice at national, local and family level. Reassertion of these rights is often necessary and in the UK the 'Patients' Charter' can be seen as one example. Bureaucratic organisa- tions such as the Health Service need certain checks or curbs to ensure their values remain egalitarian and democratic. The Health Promotion movement also epitomises this reaction to overpowering political and at times professional dominance.

Although there are certain policies which would prevent ill health there are also supreme values which may be seen to conflict with these. Obviously, banning cigarette smoking would effect better health across the nation and deaths from cardio-vascular and neoplastic conditions would probably be reduced for this generation to a noticeable degree, but much more dramatically for the next. Govern- ments resist because this would impose restriction and be counter to individual freedom. It would also reduce their revenue through taxation and prolong the life of those of pensionable age and those perceived as unproductive. However, the conflict is uncomfortable for many who see people inflicting themselves and others with dangerous cigarette smoke. The degree of acceptable restriction is open to debate – public transport and public places are now mostly non-smoking environments and such policies may become even more prevalent. Smokers' freedom has only really been limited on the basis of harm to others, evidence on the harm of passive smoking helping to provide more justification.

This conflict pervades health care. Those who provide care certainly consider they have helpful knowledge and those who approach them for help must also believe this to at least some extent. However, the perception of people outside the system may not be taken into account. For instance, those who are homeless, needy and apparently disrespectful of the mores of the system may get a rather poor reception in clinics or casualty departments. Because they are often transitory and lack any registration number, care may be denied to them. Alternate services may be provided to accommodate this way of life but in most countries there are sections of the population, admittedly varying in size, who are unable to receive services or who consider the services are too remote or irrelevant. Their values and ways of life may be too far removed from those of organised services, their independence of view may be too contrasting, making the health carers' goals of self-care and planning for the future irrelevant.

Dealing with contrasting values and cultures, appreciating what this means in practice and resisting the temptation by health carers to become resentful is essential. However, exploitation of negative reactions and the prejudice underlying them should be the focus for more education and a reorientation for any provision must reflect the needs and preferences of multiple types of consumers. In 1992, the 'Patients' Charter' was seen to reflect a more consumer-oriented service. This does provide official support for the health promotion movement and can be cited as a public document aimed explicitly to reorganise the rights of consumers and tailor care to suit them.

At all levels of international collaboration, national policy, local community networks and at the individual level, the health promotion orientation can therefore be applied. The philosophy assumes that people will have more influence on health care provision and be presented with more information, but not in a way which infers that professionals or staff have all the answers or necessarily 'knows best'. Paternalism and beneficence have been important values in the past but only the latter is still robust as a guiding principle in all we do since no member of the caring professions should harm or cause distress.

Research and health promotion

The extent to which health promotion is affecting practice or health is open to question and therefore research. It is now timely to attempt to review research which represents the full range of approaches and interventions within this movement. As the philosophical debates and semantic clarification emerge empirical work has become more possible. For instance, Patient and Health Education may be seen as components of this approach. What was labelled 'health education' has perhaps benefited from a decade of research-assessing approaches from media campaigns and advertising. This has served to alert some to the dangers of subliminal persuasion and the publication of health messages which do not respect freedom of action and decision. These approaches are discussed in this book and most now accept that raising awareness of various issues is insufficient to encourage reflection or real motivation to adopt 'healthy' behaviour. Raising public awareness through dissemination of relevant information is generally acceptable as this reflects a fundamental right of all to have access to this resource to make choices. General public knowledge that AIDS is a growing problem is clear testimony to the fact that information can be transmitted. However, much investigation is required before it is known whether risky practices are reduced as a consequence.

At all levels of practice a questioning and open approach is essential to evaluate the effects on participants. Community action and self-help groups, discussed by many contributors, may provide invaluable support for those in need but they also reflect the fact that professionals are not required to 'organise' or necessarily provide input. Both the process of establishing such a group as well as the support it provides are seen as positive effects. Evidence of this is cited in several chapters.

Emphasis on life and health at the community level and on targeting those groups in need of particular services is represented in many writings. Reforms of nursing education in the UK clearly reflect that nurses of the future need to understand social and demographic factors in order to plan appropriate strategies. Strengths within community nursing traditions will also hopefully help to influence hospital nursing. Family orientation, flexibility of working patterns with varying environmental constraints and the ability to mobilise supporting resources according to need can be seen as crucial to progressive nursing wherever it takes place. The focus on studying health within the community and mapping patterns of change through careful analysis could lead on to quite systematic research evaluations. More effort to adjust methods of working in multidisciplinary teams to accommodate change could also be made in established systems.

Examples of how this is done under crisis situations in many countries may provide valuable lessons for others. Some of the third world community initiatives described in this volume might well help to refocus some more established support services.

Increasingly writers on health promotion are now able to explain what this means in practice. This leads on to careful description of what can be done and the extent that this helps to achieve goals. Perhaps one of the most challenging arenas of all is the hospital setting, the very nexus of what is somewhat euphemistically called health care. As acute and emergency medical and nursing care has dominated the vision and expenditure of so many health services, the extent to which health promotion is encouraged and operationalised is open to research. An understanding of how practice or delivery of care can enhance the autonomy and satisfaction of consumers is gradually emerging among authors. Researchers and nurse practitioners might share the perspectives that participation in decision-making and negotiation of treatment plans are fundamental to health promotion in any setting. This is only possible in most situations where information is constantly provided and communications are open and encourage discussion and confident questioning by all involved. In the Western world this has gradually filtered through as a desirable health care climate. Staff may advocate such a policy but the next vital stage is to provide evidence that such partnership, family involvement, holistic or total care can be observed in operation. There is no clearer example of where research is needed to provide guidance for such a radical change in practice.

3 The ethics of health education

Alastair V. Campbell

Since the time of Socrates – who declared that 'the unexamined life is not worth living' and was condemned to death for the sentiment! – ethics has always been rightly regarded as a *critical* discipline. Being critical is not the same as being judgemental. The latter implies a superior stance in which the questioner knows how fallacious or erroneous the views of her opponents are. To be critical is to be a genuine questioner, one who is unsure of the answer but believes that there are real uncertainties to be explored. It is in this critical, not judgemental, spirit that I wish to explore the moral ambiguities in the current enthusiasm for health promotion.

One must concede that health promotion is an easy target for criticism, because (for the most part) it is so public that we all have views about it – indeed must be so if it is to succeed. Thus we all become critics of some health promotional campaigns merely by being members of our modern media dominated society. Many other areas of health care, by contrast, although perhaps still more morally ambiguous, are partly or wholly concealed from public scrutiny. Only when special enquiries are made as the result of some complaint or scandal do these ambiguities emerge into the light of day. So, it might be felt unfair that health promotion suffers more criticism merely because it is more visible. Against this I shall argue that health promotion contains within its own inherent logic the *demand* that it be criticised. To fail to criticise it is to fail to understand what its fundamental aims are, aims related to the fostering of a society in which there is a genuine sharing of power.

In the critical sections which follow I shall be seeking answers to the following questions: (i) how well based in fact are health promotion programmes?; (ii) are the ends achieved genuine components of health and well-being?; (iii) are the methods employed morally justified?; (iv) are the claimed benefits equitably distributed? In a short epilogue I shall discuss in a more general way the relationship between health, power and nursing.

Health promotion and the logic of science

Clearly health promotion encompasses a wide range of activities, ranging from advice and support to individuals in health care settings, through educational and advertising programmes aimed at specific groups or more generally to whole populations, and on to attempts to create a more healthy environment through social and legislative change. What all these activities have in common, however, is the assumption that a causal link has been established between a given change in the behaviour of individuals or in social conditions and an increase in health either of those individuals or of society as a whole. The term health *promotion* implies certainty about the need for such specific changes. Herein lies the difficulty, for the logic of science is not one of deductive certainty but one of inductive probability, and we are quite accustomed to finding that yesterday's scientific fact is tomorrow's scientific fallacy. But how can you promote something and emphasise its uncertainty at the same time? Of course, this problem is not unique to health promotion. It dogs the delivery of curative interventions also. But the question of factual grounding is a really critical one for health promotion, since the changes it seeks are on such a large scale and depend so heavily on mass persuasion. It is much easier for the conscientious health practitioner to warn the patient of uncertainty of outcome than for the health campaigner to lace her own campaign with a dash of doubt.

This difficulty has been explored by a number of writers. In a provocative paper published in the *Journal of Medical Ethics* Skrabanek has argued that preventive medicine exists in an 'ethical vacuum', free from the constraints which are imposed upon experimentation in other fields of medicine. Questioning the efficacy of some mass screening programmes for coronary heart disease and for breast and cervical cancer, Skrabanek (1990, p. 188) states: 'We should not confuse "prevention" with "hopes of prevention". Uncovering problems for which there is no effective treatment is not preventive medicine but a medical contribution to ill-health.' O'Hagan (1991) in an article stressing the need for fully informed consent to participation in screening and other health promotional programmes makes a similar point about the uncertainty of much that has been promoted as effective in this field. One of his examples is the poorly founded belief that lowering cholesterol will reduce mortality, in view of the recent finding that aggregate, non-cardiac deaths were higher in the intervention group than in the group who had no lipid lowering interventions. O'Hagan argues that more honesty is required both about uncertainties and about the risks associated with some intervention programmes. His conclusion is a somewhat pessimistic one: 'If our community perceives that we have been less than honest in these promotions the backlash will be formidable. On the other hand, mass informed consent may well limit recruitment and the ultimate success of such programmes (p. 123).'

Skrabanek's and O'Hagan's criticisms are largely directed at one aspect of health promotion, where mass screening techniques are employed together with medical interventions (such as lipid lowering drugs or drugs for hypertension) designed to prevent or reduce the incidence of disease. But in a review published in the *Bulletin of Medical Ethics* Sonja Hunt (1992) directs a swingeing attack on the whole promotional enterprise on grounds that it ignores the most significant scientific evidence about the causes of ill health. Hunt's paper raises a number of broader issues to which I shall return in my concluding sections, but for the present we may note her claim that health promotional activities which focus on changing individual behaviour (such as smoking, diet and exercise) are weakly founded in scientific fact and ignore the most consistent of all findings about the causes of ill health: 'The most persistent and consistent finding in studies of morbidity and mortality rates is that of a clear gradient of declining health with declining socio-economic status. This association has endured across generations and is found in every country where the necessary data have been gathered (p. 25).'

It would be a pity if we allowed the strictures of Skrabanek, O'Hagan and Hunt on inaccurate claims and skewed priorities to obscure the many well-based connections between individual behaviour and ill health. Obvious examples are the relationship between smoking and lung cancer (and other diseases), between unsafe sex or needle sharing and AIDS, and between failure to wear a seat belt and traumatic injury in car accidents. But a catalogue of certainties or near certainties will not meet the fundamental point of the critique. In every application of science there may well be a compromise, whereby we substitute a high probability with an alleged certainty. The compromise becomes more morally troubling the wider we seek to apply the science. In health promotion we are often seeking to bring about massive changes in social attitudes, in individual lifestyles, and in the regulatory framework of our society. With such goals in mind, we should make very sure not to conceal the uncertainties and be willing to have every aspect of the programmes subject to public scrutiny. If this decreases effectiveness, it may well be the moral price we have to pay for being true to the science of our endeavour.

Promotion to what end?

The next uncertainty which faces us is the definition of the end towards which all this activity aspires. To say that health promotion seeks to promote 'health' gets us no further, since few will agree how such a broad and value laden concept is to be circumscribed. In reality health promotion has to seek one or more relatively easily defined objectives, which, it is assumed, make up part of that whole we call 'health': a seat belt campaign will seek to reduce injury and death from road traffic accidents, a safe sex campaign to reduce the spread of AIDS, and so on. Yet we are bound to feel dissatisfied with this approach. With the famous WHO definition of health in mind, we might hope to promote not merely the absence of disease or disability but active well-being in various dimensions of our personal and social lives. We can easily imagine a society (we live in almost such a one) in which accidents and diseases are averted with great efficiency, but ill health is rampant. Yet how are we to define clear objectives for health promotion of this broader kind?

We may gain some clues about how to do this by considering a distinction drawn by Victoria Grace (1990) between consumerism and empowerment. Grace points out that much health promotional literature seems imbued with a language of control very similar to the quasi-military language of marketing – 'campaigning', 'targeting', 'strategising', 'evaluating', etc. Within this market ideology the consumer is given an illusion of choice, but this is firmly set within a carefully premodelled range of options defined by the promotional campaign. When this logic of consumerism is applied to health promotion we find that the human body is treated as though it were

> some kind of mechanised accessory that we can control with uncanny efficiency – an invitation to diet, exercise, practise safe sex, do numerous tests and self examinations . . . The goal would seem to be that we can incite our bodies to act with a regulated moderation entirely free from the irritating neuroses which seem to get in the way of most rational health enhancing behaviours.

I strongly agree with Grace that we need to counter this 'logic of consumerism' with a 'logic of empowerment'. The former is manipulative, the application of external power or influence: the latter is facilitative, the fostering of the individual's own complex and at times contradictory wishes. The market approach seeks to standardise needs and choices: the empowerment approach respects diversity and aims to create social conditions in which an individual's aspirations can be fulfilled, at least in part.

Can we move from this very general statement of an approach to specific objectives for health promotion? The objectives are not all that hard to define, but finding methods of achieving them may well be. For example, health promotion activities directed at young people should ideally do more than frighten them into giving up smoking, into practising safe sex or into avoiding drink driving. Our objectives should be directed at self-esteem, at an ability to form supportive relationships and at a sense of value in one's own life and one's future. But these inner changes are crucially dependent upon external conditions, such as housing, employment and educational opportunities. Thus the attempt to broaden our approach in health promotion leads us inevitably into the socio-political arena. I shall return to this point at the conclusion of this chapter.

On the devil and the good tunes

The remark, 'Why should the devil have all the good tunes?' widely attributed to General Booth was apparently made by one, the Reverend Rowland Hill. Whatever its source, it seems apposite for our next question — are the methods of health promotion morally justifiable? Since many health destructive behaviours are promoted by mass advertising, is it fair and reasonable that the same methods should be used for promoting health enhancing ones?

A major attack on the concept of health promotion as mere 'slick salesmanship' has been launched by Gill Williams (1984). For Williams health can be improved only by genuinely educational activities: 'Health promotion, like advertising campaigns, cannot hope to do more than induce superficial change, which is susceptible to the next round of gimmicks or hard sell. Longterm commitment to sensible health behaviour . . . is needed if we are to improve health (p. 194).' But the distinction between education and promotion may not be as absolute as Williams seeks to make it. I have examined this question in some detail in a chapter in Doxiadis (1990), *Ethics in Health Education*. The issue is not so much one of superficiality, as Williams suggests, for, some forms of value promotion can produce quite profound change, as Sargant (1957) documented long ago in his classic study of brainwashing and conversion techniques, *Battle for the Mind*. Rather the crucial difference is that education encourages independent thought, while some forms of promotion of values — political indoctrination and subliminal advertising are two examples — seek to bypass the hearer's capacity for critical judgment. The philosopher R. M. Hare (1972) describes the difference well: 'The educator is waiting and hoping all the time for those whom he is educating to start thinking . . . The indoctrinator, on the other hand, is watching for signs of trouble, and ready to intervene to suppress it when it appears.' There is no reason why we should not use the most attractive and professional methods available to 'sell' health values, provided we are doing it in a way that serves the end of involving the individual in a critical evaluation of what we are promoting. This proviso, however, does mean that some tunes we must leave only to the devil! There are some telling examples from anti-smoking advertisements. A Western Australian TV ad 'Pretty Face' depicts the metamorphosis of a young woman's face into an old hag with foul breath – the message is one which depends for its appeal on the ageist and sexist messages of much media advertising. A British ad 'Kathy' plays on the fears which children have that their parents who smoke will die. The punchline is 'If you won't give up smoking for yourself, do it for your kids'. Other examples entail warning smokers of the outcomes of peripheral vascular disease in gangrene and amputation of a limb. The stress on disfigurement again buys into the dominant attitudes of a culture which finds the disabled an embarassment.

But – you may ask – why be so purist about the methods employed, if the disgust or fear which they create can pull people up short and make them think more carefully about their actions? Several other arresting ads will no doubt come to mind – such as the Australian 'Grim Reaper' AIDS ad or the drink-drive scenarios set in accident emergency rooms. We are confronted here with a familiar and age old debate in ethics – does the end justify the means? To find an answer we need to remember that the end we seek is not simply a statistical reduction in smokers, or drunk drivers, or AIDS sufferers. These are, of course, highly desirable objectives, but there has been no gain in promoting health if the conditions which produced these destructive outcomes remain unchanged. We *may* be able to scare people out of some risky behaviour but we cannot scare them into health, especially when much that brings the ill health is not within their control. Thus an approach to health promotion which merely picks on the obvious targets and which uses the culture's own health denying values to try to change behaviour has lost sight of the end in a preoccupation with one quite restricted range of means, the seductive techniques of the 'hidden persuaders'.

On promoting equity

My critique of some of the methods of health promotion leads me back to the point made by Sonja Hunt in her review article, that much health promotional activity ignores the most obvious of all the causes of ill health – social inequality. Indeed, as Hunt also observes, health promotion in its 'targeting' mode can be a powerful way of diverting attention from this root cause. The poor have only themselves to blame, it would seem, if they turn to smoking, alcohol and other drugs, unprotected sex and unhealthy food. The fervour of some health campaigns is reminiscent of the evangelical appeals of a previous age –

'yield not to temptation' – all that society's misfits required was a change of heart – turn to Jesus . . . or to healthy lifestyles.

The history of health promotion is, of course, quite different from such an apolitical, individualistic stance. The public health movement was essentially and inevitably one of radical social reform. The rich and the powerful had to be persuaded to do something about the appalling conditions of the poor and about the insanitary state of the inner cities – if for no other reason than that it was in their long-term self-interest to do so. Perhaps the dramatic improvements in public health over this century have blinded us to the need to keep social change firmly on the agenda of health promotion. Although the overall health of the nation has steadily risen over the decades, the correlation between health and social class remains as firm as ever. Ill health dogs the poor. Thus health promotion must mean structural, not merely individual change.

How can this aspect of health promotion be relevant to people in the health professions? Surely structural change is a task for politicians or for voluntary associations and pressure groups. How can one both be in a structure (at quite an advantageous level) and change that structure at the same time? Not necessarily. The answer lies in a proper understanding of the nature of a profession. There have been strong moves in our time to seek to reduce the professional ideal to mere rhetoric, concealing the pursuit of monopolistic power. 'Professions', it is argued, are no different from other occupations, and their claim to a special ethic is merely a device to keep their activities free from outside interference. In my book, *Moderated Love* (Campbell, 1984), I have tried to redefine the vocational aspect of professional care, while acknowledging the realities of the professions' pursuit of power and self-interest. There will always be an ambiguity between altruism and egoism in professional care, but nevertheless a spontaneous and open-ended commitment to the good of the other remains a vital part of the professional relationship. Included within this vocational element is what I have called the 'prophetic role' of the professions. Because they are in a unique position to see the outcomes of the health destructive aspects of our society, they have a special responsibility to publicise these and to seek to have them changed. A profession cannot fulfil its ideals merely by focusing on the individual patient: it must ask radical questions about the social origins of ill health.

Thus those health professionals who become involved in health promotion need to ask questions about the distribution of benefit which their efforts bring. To what extent is health promotion merely reinforcing the status quo, the greatest beneficiaries being those who are already well able to cater for their own health needs, and who have the power and social influence to change things further to their own advantage? How much effort in health promotion goes into those sectors of our society where there is multiple deprivation, or where the illness carries such a social stigma that it is quietly ignored? Which health promotion activities give the means to people to change their own health prospects, rather than merely reducing the grosser effects of their disadvantaged status? Where is the main research effort directed? Where do the big budgets cluster – round the needs of the poorest in our society or round the worries of the affluent? These are the questions about equity in health promotion which a truly critical ethical appraisal must ask. And because these are questions which concern our whole society, not the private and confidential questions of the individual patient, they need to be asked publicly and unapologetically by those who see their task to be that of not only the care of the sick, but the promotion of the health of all in our society. They need to be asked by professionals who see the outcomes of these injustices on individual lives.

Epilogue – health and power

I come finally to the relevance of all this to health promotion in nursing. I suggest that we can best understand this in terms of the relationship between heath and power. For I believe that nursing has always had an interesting and at times quite ambivalent relationship to power. I am sure I do not need to rehearse the pilgrimage of the nursing profession from the mixed images of slattern and nun, through the starched and pure 'handmaiden' of the doctor, to today's era of a quite confident and increasingly independent profession. It is a story of the gradual evolution of a different kind of power from that of the medical profession. In contrast with the interventionist and episodic nature of the medical relationship, the nurse's professionalism consists more in sustaining presence and in the facilitation of the patient's own coping abilities. These features of nursing have led me to describe it as 'skilled companionship' (Campbell, 1984), the nurse being one of the people who helps the patient to journey on – to independent life or to a peaceful death. The power which the nurse possesses is thus of quite a subtle kind, different from the death defying power so often falsely ascribed to the doctor. The power of nursing, when rightly used, is one which knows when to hold and support without possessiveness, and when to motivate and let go, without bullying or rejection.

Another way of describing the nature of nursing makes its relationship to health promotion quite obvious – it is, or should be, a caring which empowers the patient. Thus all good nursing is a form of health promotion. It helps the other person mobilise inner resources to deal with the illness or disability and to find those resources which allow the self to resume control. The question for the nursing profession is whether this quiet and often overlooked form of power can find a voice to be heard that will ensure that health promotion is genuine empowerment of the dispossessed and vulnerable. Will this research find formulations that really help us to promote health rather than tinkering with the symptoms? Can the profession break the narrow bounds of an individualistic ethic and help us all to confront the social origins of ill health? Have nurses got stories to share with each other that show how their skills will translate not only into solace for the sick but into gains for the healthy. Even if these stories are of trying such things and failing, there is much that society should learn from the new professionalism in nursing.

So, it would be good to think that in making health promotion an important theme for nursing, the profession was taking a *risk*. This would suggest to me that nurses are not just (as we all so often are) just 'dedicated followers of fashion' but that they realised, as Socrates did, that when ethics intersects with politics you are heading for the hemlock!

References

Campbell, A. V. (1984). *Moderated Love*. SPCK: London, chapter 3.
Campbell, A. V. (1990). Education or indoctrination? The issue of autonomy in health education, in Doxiadis, S. (ed.). *Ethics in Health Education*. John Wiley: Chichester.
Chapman, S. (1988). For debate: the means/ends problem in health promotion. *Medical Journal of Australia, 149*, 256–60.
Doxiadis S. (1990). *Ethics in Health Education*. John Wiley, Chichester.
Grace. V. (1990). Orienting health promotion strategies. Paper presented at First Annual Conference of Health Promotion Forum for New Zealand, Auckland (unpublished).
Hare, R. M. (1972) in Snook, I. A. (ed.). *Concepts of Indoctrination*. Routledge: London.
Hunt, S. (1992). Prevention health promotion and social inequalities. *Bulletin of Medical Ethics* (May), 25.
O'Hagan, J. (1991). The ethics of informed consent in relation to prevention screening programmes. *New Zealand Medical Journal, 27* (March), 123.
Sargent, W. W. (1957). *Battle for the Mind*. Heinemann: London.
Skrabanek, P. (1990). Why is preventive medicine exempted from ethical constraints? *Journal of Medical Ethics, 16*, 188.
Williams, G. (1984). Health promotion – caring concern or slick salesmanship? *Journal of Medical Ethics, 10*, 191–5.

4 Health promotion – a human science?

Alan Cribb

The idea of health promotion

It is worth saying a few words about the meaning of health promotion. Even if the concept of health was straightforward, the idea of health promotion would still be puzzling not least because of its apparent boundlessness. It does not refer to any specific set of professional roles or institutional settings, and therefore cannot be defined or delimited in that way. It cannot even be delimited by reference to a larger set of deliberate *activities*, not only because it would be difficult to know which activities are not connected to health, but also because some processes which are, in one way or another, unintended can be seen to promote or undermine health. To put it a little abstractly, health promotion denotes a conceptual space rather than a clear professional policy or institutional domain; and it is a space of debate, uncertainty and ambiguity. This elasticity makes it a fruitful expression for reconceptualising health care and health education, but it also makes it useful for rhetorical and ideological purposes.

Some of the health promotion literature discusses appropriate means and ends for health education and health promotion in terms of the relative benefits of competing models. Indeed there are now a number of meta-analyses which review the models literature (Caplan and Holland, 1990; French, 1990; Beattie, 1991). One of the strengths of this literature is that it covers both issues of principle and what might be called 'technical' issues. Thus the models based discussion of what is 'best' is not only about what is morally and politically acceptable but also about what is 'effective'. But this can also be a weakness. There is the risk of fudging together the two kinds of issues so that neither can be seen clearly. So that, for instance, it is sometimes not clear whether the 'self-empowerment' model is being advocated because it is thought to be 'effective' at promoting health (under some conception) or because it respects individual autonomy. Is self-empowerment supposed to refer to the means or the end of health promotion? This relates to the classic concern of the reflective practitioner, 'In the last resort am I aiming for "compliance" or informed choice?' For this reason I want to begin by clearly separating out the technical issues and the ethical issues, even though this involves oversimplification and distortion. This separation also relates to a tension in the literature of health promotion between what might be called health promotion as behavioural science and health promotion as care.

Behavioural science or care?

A substantial part of the health promotion literature is made up of 'scientific papers' published in academic and professional journals. These papers commonly employ experimental, quasi-experimental and statistical methods. Often these are aimed at understanding the processes of and/or measuring the effectiveness of interventions. Sometimes they are explicitly aimed at developing and testing theories of 'health behaviour'. It is part of conventional (although not universal) wisdom that to proceed 'scientifically' is to proceed under the flag of one or another such theory. Hence health promotion can be seen as behavioural science; it draws upon, and contributes to, social sciences particularly psychology and social psychology. Its students are familiar with such things as the health belief model (and its refinements) and the theory of reasoned action, and their use to help explain and predict 'health behaviour' and the relative success or failure of interventions (Bennett and Hodgson, 1992). This literature falls squarely into the positivistic tradition. Inquiry is seen as the means to gain 'technical control' over the objects of knowledge, in this case other human beings (Habermas, 1966). By gaining a clear picture of the causes of behaviour the professional 'technocrats' can modify interventions so as to optimise the probability of achieving the desired outcome (Fay, 1987).

This behavioural science picture of health promotion makes is sound highly manipulative, but it is often said that all 'scientific knowledge' can be both used and abused. The question, some might argue, is whether or not any such knowledge is used responsibly and directed toward good ends. This takes us on to the second set of health promotion literature – the literature about ethics and principles. The simple fact that health promotion sometimes entails uninvited interference in the lives of well people raises ethical issues. These issues and others have always been of concern to the professional community and they have slowly won attention from academic ethicists (Doxiadis, 1987; Wikler, 1987). Even more influential, however, has been the attention given to issues of principle by the WHO in its articulation and advocacy of the concept of health promotion. WHO has been partly responsible for the idea that certain values are intrinsic to health promotion including participation and equality (WHO, 1986). Indeed the use of 'health promotion' as a normative expression to mean, in part, a morally approved form of health management has become quite common. There is disagreement as to what the moral content is, much of it about ideology and the proper scope of individualistic analyses, but the need to conceive of health promotion normatively is not in doubt (Dines and Cribb, 1993). At the heart of this literature is the picture of health promotion as dialogue and collaboration between all parties, including the objects of health promotion, who are thereby transformed into subjects.

If we consider these two parts of the literature together the tension between them is obvious. The former sees human beings under the description of behavioural models and generalisations. Just as we learn tricks to get our pets to take their medicine we can learn the scientific 'tricks' of promoting human health. We can learn which buttons to press, which strings to pull, to get results, or more precisely to increase the chance of getting results. The latter sees human beings first and foremost as individuals with the capacity of autonomy, and worthy of respect as 'ends in themselves' and (to complete the slogan derived from Kant) 'not merely as means to an end'. Closely associated with this tension is the endless debate about how far it is possible to operate with 'objective', expert conceptions of health as opposed to more subjective and 'subject-centred' conceptions.

Health promotion as humane science

One way forward is to see if these two pictures can be added together. The differences between them have been exaggerated in the form in which they have been presented here. It might be better to look at them as complementary, as contributing equally valid but qualitatively different types of insight. Something like this is seemingly essential for any 'caring profession' or 'human science'. Generalisation and reductionism have to be combined with a holism that includes respect for the individual and the particular. This challenge is not unique to health promotion and others have to handle this dialectic.

Superficially it may seem that these pictures can be related by seeing the 'behavioural science' as about means and the 'care' as about ends. It is often said that science cannot determine ends so it is tempting to settle on this division of labour. This would entail a good deal of consultation and negotiation in setting objectives, but then the professionals would take responsibility for choosing the most effective methods to meet them. However, a moments thought shows that, in principle, no simple division of labour will do. The distinction between means and ends breaks down as soon as we allow ethical considerations into the analysis. For our 'ends' (such as autonomy or equality) have to be respected as we act, and not just in the goals we cite to justify acting.

There are notorious philosophical problems in reconciling positivistic and humanistic perspectives; but it is important to try to understand how technical issues and ethical issues relate together. In this context ethics cannot be seen merely as an 'add-on', as a way of making technology more palatable. In this picture health professionals decide 'what is for the best' and then attempt to make it morally acceptable. Open-minded ethical debate will necessarily challenge the values built into interventions and their legitimacy. Hence the 'classic concern' referred to above:

> Am I using the language and the skills of 'self-empowerment' to try to make someone change their behaviour? Is that my real objective though it may be hidden (even from myself)? Am I treating someone with respect and encouraging their participation because this allows more subtle and possibly more effective forms of manipulation?

I do not wish to suggest a clear-cut condemnation of this behaviour. Of course, it is possible to make out an ethical case for forms of paternalism, and even for coercion where there is potentially a great gain in welfare. The worry is that sometimes these values are simply assumed as part of a technical attitude to work.

This takes me to the crux of what I want to say. From a philosophical point of view ethics cannot be treated as a mere 'add-on' to techniques of manipulation, but in practice the *language* of ethics and principles can be used in precisely this way. It can operate as a veneer of respectability, as public relations, as a way of legitimating dubious practice, and as a smokescreen to obscure real ethical issues. As ever the difference between theory and practice stems from the fact that reality is not simply a product of reason or rational agency. We can produce theories of health behaviour, theories of ethics, and models of health promotion, and debate their respective merits. But we cannot distil the real world of 'health promotion' from them. In reality all of the things which are done under the name of health promotion will be done as one element in, and under the conditions of, the existing institutions and cultures of health care or public policy. In other words, once having recognised that there is a tension between the languages of 'behavioural science' and the languages of 'care', it is not enough simply to be in favour of the latter. It is not enough to say that human sciences should first be human, and that this is a sufficient corrective for the scientific value of technical control. Whilst this may be arguable at an academic level (it would be disputed), to take this line is to ignore the ways in which talk of care or human values are often a mask for exercise of professional power.

Health promotion as a technology of control

Given the critical and sceptical tone of this discussion, I might as well adopt the idiom of that most celebrated anti-guru of postmodernism, Michel Foucault (1979). This will enable me to come at the same issues from a slightly different angle, and to set out (and perhaps exaggerate) the potential dangers of health promotion. What is distinctive in Foucault's analysis is his exploration of the many ways in which patterns of social 'knowledge' are intimately interconnected with patterns of power. The possibilities of health promotion are determined by patterns of power in which certain groups are dominant. The targets set by the government, the priorities of senior managers and professionals, the systems of resourcing, and favoured academic perspectives such as epidemiology and health economics shape the reality of health promotion more than any normative conception of what it ought to be.

From this point of view the policies and practices of health promotion are not best understood as the outcome of disinterested professional judgement and autonomy, but rather as an aspect of criss-crossing systems of social regulation and control. However well intentioned, and however much they may be dressed up as forms of care or social justice, health promotion activities inevitably embody forms of domination. This is not to say that there is some monolithic system of control; rather forms of power may be small scale or local, they may relate chiefly to certain groups or issues, and they may reinforce one another or conflict. The basic framework of a Foucauldian analysis of power and social control can be set out in a few sentences, and in so doing its relevance to health promotion is striking (Turner, 1987; Ball, 1990).

According to Foucault the human sciences are allied to, and closely interwoven with, professional groups and forms of 'government'. Here 'government' does not simply refer to the exercise of macropolitical power but encompasses less overt or deliberate, and more subtle forms of control. Typically these forms of government are built into relations of 'power-knowledge' in which those 'in the know' monitor those who are not. This 'surveillance' acts as a technology of control irrespective of the intentions of professionals because it embodies standards of good and bad, and it brings them into the public domain and into the self-consciousness of the governed. Indeed the strength of these power relations resides in large part from the fact that ultimately they rest upon 'self-government' and 'self-control'. Systems of appraisal provide a clear example. It is possible to have one's work appraised in a supportive and constructive environment; it is not uncommon for these procedures to be based around self-appraisal and for a lot of emphasis to be placed upon autonomy and empowerment. Yet despite this emphasis, *or because of it*, appraisal acts as a very effective mechanism for bringing individuals into line with the objectives of their employing institution. There are always forms of resistance but it is sometimes easier to resist a blunter instrument.

Health promotion fits only too neatly into this framework. It relates to all aspects and facets of life and lifestyle. The emphasis on prevention encourages continuous monitoring of the well in addition to the sick. The call for health promotion to become a part of every sector, including all parts of the health service, means that there are to be multiple sites for surveillance. All of these factors suggest that holism can be a double-edged sword. Finally, as we have seen, the 'scientific' literature makes explicit use of such things as 'subjective norms' and 'self-regulation' as part of the technology of health promotion (Bennett and Hodgson, 1992).

There are many who are sceptical about political power distorting the philosophy of health promotion. This has been a common response to *The Health of the Nation* (DOH, 1992). Similarly, there is some scepticism about the potential of health promotion in primary health care being diminished by patterns of funding that might support medicalisation and reinforce inequities (Waller *et al.*, 1990; Smith, 1991). These are related examples of concerns about government and social control. If we take a Foucauldian analysis seriously we should be equally sceptical about more personal and homely interventions, and the extent to which they involve 'government' (Bloor and McIntosh, 1990). It might even be said that we should look particularly closely at those interventions that are legitimised by talk of 'participation' or 'empowerment'. These ideas, which are meant to be incompatible with professional domination, can also be used to oil the new mechanisms of social control.

References

Ball, S. (ed.) (1990). *Foucault and Education*, Routledge: London.

Beattie, A. (1991). Knowledge and control in health promotion: a test case for social policy and social theory, in Gabe, J., Calnan, M., and Bury, M. (eds). *The Sociology of the Health Service*. Routledge: London.

Bennett, P. and Hodgson, R. (1992). Psychology and health promotion, in Bunton, R. and Macdonald, G. (eds). *Health Promotion – Disciplines and Diversity*. Routledge: London.

Bloor, M., and McIntosh, J. (1990). Surveillance and concealment: a comparison of techniques of client resistance in therapeutic communities and health visiting, in Cunningham, B. S. and McKeganey, N. P. (eds). *Readings in Medical Sociology.* Routledge: London.

Caplan, R. and Holland, R. (1990). Rethinking health education theory. *Health Education Journal, 49,* 1.

Dines, A. and Cribb, A. (1993). *Health Promotion: Concepts and Practice.* Blackwell: Oxford.

Department of Health (1992). *The Health of the Nation.* HMSO: London.

Doxiadis, S. (ed.) (1987). *Ethical Dilemmas in Health Promotion.* John Wiley: Chichester.

Fay, B. (1987). *Critical Social Science.* Polity Press: Cambridge.

Foucault, M. (1979). *Discipline and Punish.* Penguin: Harmondsworth.

French, J. (1990). Boundaries and horizons, the role of health education within health promotion. *Health Education Journal, 49,* 1.

Habermas, J. (1966). Knowledge and Interests, *Inquiry, 9,* 4.

Smith, S. (1991). Practice nurses told to question use of skills. *Nursing Times, 87,* 17.

Turner, B. (1987). *Medical Power and Social Knowledge.* Sage: London.

Waller, D., Agness, M. and Mont, D. (1990). Health checks in general practice. *British Medical Journal, 300,* 1115.

WHO (1986). Discussion document on the concepts and principles of health promotion. *Health Promotion, 1,* 1.

Wikler, D. (1987). Who should be blamed for being sick? *Health Education Quarterly, 14,* 1.

5 A social behavioural approach to understanding and promoting condom use

Janet M. Walker

Introduction

It is commonly assumed that if individuals are provided with information about serious health risks to themselves, together with actions which they can take to reduce or eliminate that risk, a sequence of cognitive events will follow which should culminate in the desired behavioural outcomes. Information about health risk may reinforce, increase or challenge existing knowledge. It is assumed that new knowledge shapes beliefs about behavioural outcomes which leads, in turn, to a shift in attitudes, the intention to change behaviour and, ultimately, to behaviour change. The Health Belief Model (HBM, Janz and Becker, 1984) and the Theory of Planned Behaviour (TPB, Ajzen, 1988) are two examples of models designed to explain and predict health-related behaviours. The HBM seeks to explain health behaviours in terms of perceived vulnerability to, and severity of the disease in question, together with the perceived benefits and barriers of taking action. The TPB predicts behavioural intentions in terms of the individual's attitude towards the required behaviour, perceived normative influences and perceived behavioural control.

A number of recent papers have cast doubt upon the predictive value of these models and have offered possible reasons for their failure. An important criticism of both theories was offered by Hunt and Martin (1988) who suggested that most health-related behaviours occur routinely (for example brushing teeth, buying and cooking food or smoking) and are not, therefore, the immediate product of rational thinking. Rutter and Calnan (1987) studied the effects of a health educational class to promote breast self-examination. Perceived vulnerability to breast cancer predicted the willingness of individuals to attend the class. However, the best predictor of both frequency and technique of breast self-examination after the course of instruction was frequency and technique prior to attendance. Bad habits, it seems, die hard while good habits, once cultivated, are likely to endure.

Further evidence of difficulties in changing both attitudes and behaviour was highlighted by Eiser and Gentle (1989) who showed that large-scale health campaigns aimed at providing information to reduce risk factors associated with coronary heart disease appealed most to those whose behaviour was least in need of change. These and similar findings are a cause of much concern to health educators who wish to reduce the risk of spread of HIV/AIDS via normal sexual activity among young people. Media reports throughout 1992 suggest the failure of campaigns to change heterosexual behaviour, although there is little evidence of lack of knowledge about the risk factors involved. Hunt and Martin (1988) suggested that mass campaigns are probably most useful in creating a climate of opinion conducive to change and in promoting the conscious awareness of habitual behaviours. However, providing information has little direct impact on behaviour.

Social processes and sexual behaviour

Ingham (1989) challenged the validity of cognitive models in predicting sexual behaviour and highlighted some of the social pressures which cause young people to engage in unprotected sexual behaviour in spite of good intentions. These include strong pressures to engage in sexual intercourse from peer group and partners. Ingham (1990) found that young women are frequently under pressure from potential sexual partners to engage in sex without a condom. He also identified that young people appear to lack the complex social skills required to negotiate condom use. Ingham has encouraged us to examine more closely the interpersonal influences on sexual behaviour, whereas models of belief-attitude-behaviour have focused upon intrapersonal (rational) processes.

Behavioural analysis of condom use

Using a condom involves planned behaviours which serve the specific purposes of preventing unwanted pregnancy and protecting against sexually transmitted diseases, including HIV/AIDS. However, as Hunt and Martin (1988) pointed out, although behaviours may be health related, health is not necessarily a primary consideration when they are being carried out. The basic principles of applied behaviour analysis suggests that a behaviour, within a particular context, is influenced by its perceived consequences which include:

- the strength of the reinforcer or punisher (this may be very subjective);
- the immediacy of the consequences;
- the certainty of the consequences;

(Reinforcers increase the likelihood of a behaviour, punishers reduce their likelihood. Reward or physical punishment is not necessarily implied.)

In *Table 5.1*, behavioural principles are used to weigh the likelihood of engaging in sexual intercourse against preserving health, assuming that, at the outset, both are regarded as equally important. It is apparent, from this analysis, that health is unlikely to be a primary motivator of sexual behaviour because health outcomes, including pregnancy, are neither immediate nor certain, while the physical and social reinforcers of sexual intercourse are both immediate and relatively certain. Thus calls for sexual abstinence *on health grounds alone* are unlikely to succeed (although other reasons may be more persuasive.

Table 5.2 uses the same principles to compare protected with unprotected sex. The outcomes of each are equally immediate, although the outcomes of using a condom may be rather less certain because of the social and practical skills involved. In addition to this, the strength of the reinforcement of condom use may be reduced not

Table 5.1 *Behavioural analysis of sex versus health outcomes*

	Sex	Health
1. Strength of positive consequences	+++	+++
2. Immediacy of the consequences	+++	−
3. Certainty of the consequences	++	−

+++ strong influence − no influence

Table 5.2 *Behavioural analysis of sex with or without a condom*

	Condom use: with	without
1. Strength of positive consequences	++	+++
2. Immediacy of the consequences	+++	+++
3. Certainty of the consequences	+	++

only by a reduction of sensation, but difficulties in negotiating use, particularly when sex is taking place with a relatively unfamiliar partner. These factors appear to reduce the probability that individuals will choose to use condoms, particular in those situations where they are most needed.

Social behaviour and social influences on behaviour

It is often forgotten that one of the most important universal reinforcers or punishers of any behaviour which takes place in a social setting is likely to be the social approval or disapproval of other people, whether expressed verbally or non-verbally. We are socialised, throughout childhood, to respond to the approval and disapproval of our parents, teachers and peer group. This is partially reflected in the 'subjective norm' referred to by Ajzen (1988), although social reinforcers or punishers are probably far more ubiquitous than any conscious consideration of 'what those who matter to me think I should do'. Approval or disapproval is generally the expression of an attitude or cultural value. In fact, the chief importance of attitudes, which is frequently overlooked, is that they are not merely private events but public expressions of socially constructed beliefs and values, generally expressed verbally or non-verbally in terms of approval or disapproval. My behaviour is much more likely to be influenced by *your* attitudes than my own. In other words, perceived social desirability is an extremely powerful reinforcer of punisher of human behaviour.

Figure 5.1 offers a cognitive model in which the important function of attitudes is the production of expressive, rather than goal-directed, behaviours. The attitudes of one person may exert a reinforcing or punishing influence upon the goal-directed behaviour of another person. More important, the combined attitudes and opinions of a group of individuals can be very effective in changing or maintaining the voluntary behaviour of any individual who shares similar cultural values and norms. Figure 5.3 illustrates *one element* in a dynamic process in which the expressive behaviour of one individual, or group of individuals directly influences the deliberate voluntary behaviours of another individual or group of individuals. The expressed attitudes of one individual or group also draw to conscious attention those observable habitual behaviours of another individual or group which are deemed to be socially undesirable.

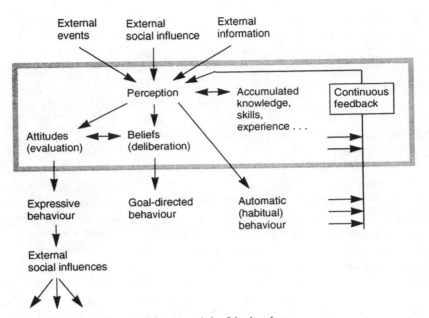

Figure 5.1 *Social cognitive model of behaviour*

Mass appeal

One of the best ways of reaching a wide audience is through the mass media, while the most effective way of influencing people to use a particular product is through marketing and advertising aimed at the right target audience. Behavioural principles suggest that, while condoms are unlikely to be used by young people for purely health reasons, the increased certainty of immediate reinforcement from having and using a product with high social desirability and approval would increase its purchase and use. A product which is available in plain packages from chemists shops, toilets or free from family planning centres is hardly likely to score high on social prestige. Attempts to market condoms as fun items have so far been hampered by the production of inferior quality goods, a 'smutty' image, or severe limitations on advertising. It is suggested that the quickest way to cultivate condom use on a wide scale is to lift all advertising restrictions and market high quality condoms in the same way as a certain brand of expensive ice cream. A young person with the right 'gear' gains self-confidence. The anticipation of social approval for being 'cool' and using the right condom would ensure that the majority would comply with the new social norm in the same way that young people conform to norms for clothing and other items. As a result, the issue would cease to be 'should I use a condom?' and become 'which condom should I use?' Although it is essential that any association with soft pornography should be avoided, some degree of indignation among an older minority may actually increase the social prestige of these products among the teenage population.

Moral and ethical issues

The moral and ethical issues associated with advertising a sexual product to young people cannot be ignored. It carries with it the spectre of mass manipulation of youngsters to engage in promiscuous behaviour. However, it is necessary to ask what the difference is between advertising one product, lager, which encourages young people to consume something which frequently leads to loss of control, and another product, condoms, which is likely to offer reasonable protection against the worst outcomes (pregnancy, sexually transmitted diseases and HIV) of a normal behaviour which many young people are likely to engage in anyway. Is it morally and ethically sound deliberately to deny young people access to a type of promotional advertising which could save their lives?

Empowerment

There is an alternative approach to encouraging responsible attitudes towards sex and the use of condoms, but it is a long-term one. It involves the focus, from an early age, upon the empowerment of young people to resist social pressures, including sexual advances and advertising, and to act upon informed choices. There is evidence that the health-related behaviour of teenagers is influenced by parenting style, such that those with warm–directive (authoritative) parents are more likely to have internal locus of control and high self-esteem (Baumrind, 1967) and be able to resist pressure to smoke, drink alcohol and use solvents (Foxcroft and Lowe, 1992). There is further evidence that school education packages can enhance empowerment in children (Igoe, 1992). Education in parenting skills and empowerment education in schools may well be the best solution in the long term. The question confronting us at present is 'can we afford to wait that long?'

Summary

Health education campaigns have been generally successful in increasing knowledge and creating a climate of opinion but relatively unsuccessful, at least in the short term, in changing risky behaviour. Models of health behaviour have focused upon the intrapersonal relationship between knowledge, beliefs, attitudes and behaviour, but have ignored the interpersonal significance of expressive behaviour as a potential reinforcer or punisher of behaviour in any social context. An alternative interpersonal model of health behaviour, based upon social behavioural principles, is offered in which goal-directed and expressive behaviours are identified as serving different functions. The expressive behaviour of one individual or group is likely to exert a reinforcing or punishing influence upon the habitual or deliberate behaviour of another individual or group. Based upon this theoretical model, it is argued that the most effective way to reduce the risk of HIV/AIDS among sexually active young people, in the short term, is to market the condom as a product which will immediately increase the wearer's social prestige and ensure the reinforcing social approval of his or her social group.

References

Ajzen, I. (1988). *Attitudes, Personality and Behaviour*. Open University Press: Milton Keynes.

Baumrind, D. (1967). Child care practices anteceding three patterns of preschool behaviour. *Genetic Psychological Monographs*, 75, 43–88.

Eiser, J. R. and Gentle, P. (1989). Health beliefs and attitudes to publicity campaigns for health promotion. *Psychology and Health*, 3, 111–20.

Foxcroft, D. and Lowe, G. (1992). Family influences and health lifestyles of teenage drinkers. Paper presented at the British Psychological Society Health Psychology Section Annual Conference, St Andrews (September).

Hunt, S. M. and Martin, C. J. (1988). Health-related behaviour change – a test of a new model. *Psychology and Health*, 2, 209–30.

Igoe, J. (1992). Healthier children through empowerment. Paper given at 'Promoting Health', International Research conference for Nurses, London (September).

Ingham, R. (1989). Lay theories and models of beliefs and behaviour. *Health Psychology Update*, 4, 11–16. British Psychological Society: Leicester.

Ingham, R. (1990). Getting to know you: young people's knowledge of their partner at first sexual experience. Published Report, Department of Psychology, Southampton University.

Janz, N. K. and Becker, M. H. (1984). The health belief model: a decade later. *Health Education Quarterly*, 11, 1–47.

Rutter, D. R., and Calnan, M. (1987). Do health beliefs predict health behaviour? A further analysis of breast self-examination, in Dent, H. R. (ed.). *Clinical Psychology: Research and Development*. Croom Helm: London.

6 A case study of ethical issues in health promotion – mammography screening: the nurse's position

Alison Dines

Introduction

All nurses in the United Kingdom may be called upon to play a part in the national mammography screening programme. This may involve anything from working in a screening centre to simply being ready to inform members of the public about breast cancer screening should their professional knowledge be called upon. The programme, which forms an important part of the government's health promotion strategy, poses complex ethical issues. No work has so far examined how nurses and other health promoters might respond to these. This chapter explores the nurse's position in the light of these moral dilemmas.

Background to mammography screening

Early detection of disease through screening is generally held to be one component of health promotion (see for example Tannahill, 1985). The United Kingdom now has a national mammography screening programme for the early detection of breast cancer as part of its health promotion strategy (Department of Health, 1992). This was originally recommended by the Forrest Report in 1986 (Department of Health and Social Security, 1986). Now women between 50 and 64 years are invited to be screened every three years. The rationale for this is that successful screening will detect the disease at a stage when there is scope for effective treatment, thereby reducing the overall mortality rate.

Mammography, however, is a contentious issue. Internationally, opinion differs considerably about its benefit. Thus Sir Patrick Forrest (1990, p. 104) concluded, 'There can be no doubt that screening by mammography benefits women who develop breast cancer.' In contrast, Schmidt (1990, p. 223), an authority writing from Switzerland, believes, 'Breast cancer screening does likely more harm than good . . . to women of the 50–75 age group.' The uncertainty surrounding mammography is further complicated by the fact that the first reports from the UK programme (UK Trial of Early Detection of Breast Cancer Group, 1988), whilst demonstrating that the mortality rate *is* lower in the screened population by 15 per cent, did *not show this to be statistically significant*. The reasons for the absence of *statistical* benefit are complex, but it may be due to low attendance for mammography.

Mammography therefore raises complex ethical issues. This chapter explores the nurse's position in the light of these moral dilemmas. Two specific questions will be addressed. What position should a nurse take in a position of such uncertainty? In addition, if as health promoters we are interested in participation and enablement, how can we offer women health education in this situation?

The nurse's position

The question 'what is an ethical response in a situation of such uncertainty?' may be approached by thinking about four positions a nurse might adopt. These are outlined below.

Position I

The nurse might assess the evidence and decide mammography is of benefit and therefore be fully involved with the programme.

Position II

The nurse might assess the evidence, decide mammography is harmful, have no involvement with the programme and endeavour to have it stopped.

Position III

The nurse might decide it is best not to be involved with a programme that is not proven and wait until the evidence is conclusive.

Position IV

The nurse might decide to maintain a 'healthy scepticism' about the programme, be involved with it, whilst at the same time observing the continued evaluation of the effectiveness of the programme and informing women about the uncertain situation.

Let us now examine these positions in greater depth. Each 'position' has been given a name to help capture something of the flavour of the ethical stance being adopted.

Position I 'NURSE COMMITTED'

A nurse of this persuasion might say: *'The negative findings of various research reports into mammography screening can all be explained in terms of various methodological issues. Breast cancer is a huge problem and we must do something about it. I think time will show it to work.'*

It is interesting when examining each of these 'positions' to look at some of the assumptions being made. Nurse Committed assumes that 'doing something' in the face of a problem is better than doing nothing. This is an approach almost 'reinforced' at times by nursing itself. It has been challenged by some in recent years as not always appropriate. The advantages of Nurse Committed's approach is that women have a chance of being helped in the fight against breast cancer. In addition, mammography has the best chance of being tested as a new procedure because of high uptake. The disadvantages of her stance are that if mammography is subsequently found not to benefit women the public may be harmed through the perceived misuse of resources, a loss of confidence in health promoters and what may be viewed as an unnecessary intrusion into people's lives. The moral duties which are pertinent here are the duty of beneficence or doing good, the duty of veracity or truth telling and the duty of non-maleficence or not causing harm.

Position II 'NURSE AGIN'

A nurse of this persuasion might say: *'There is enough evidence from the international trials to show that mammography is not working. We are raising false expectations to allow it to continue. It was only introduced because it was politically useful in an election year.'*

The advantage of Nurse Agin's position is that it avoids the possibility of harming the public, at least in the short term. The disadvantage, however, is that mammography remains untested and women continue to die with breast cancer. The same moral duties of non-maleficence, veracity and beneficence mentioned with Nurse Committed are also relevant here.

Position III 'NURSE SIDELINES'

This nurse might say: *'It is unethical to offer untested remedies to members of the public. Until there is sufficient evidence to prove mammography works I cannot be involved.'*

Nurse Sidelines makes some interesting assumptions. First, that it is possible to 'prove' something. Many thinkers concerned with the philosophy of science would question this view of scientific knowledge. She also assumes it is possible to 'not be involved' and that inaction is a morally neutral position. Once again, many people would challenge this, seeing inaction as equivalent to a decision not to act and therefore not as neutral as we might first think. The advantage of Nurse Sidelines position is that she does not personally risk causing harm to members of the public through a new procedure. The disadvantage of the view is that if everyone adopted this position no advances in research would ever be made and in this case women would continue to die of breast cancer. Similar moral duties appear to be important here to those identified with Nurse Committed and Nurse Agin, in particular the tension between present and future beneficence.

Position IV 'NURSE FENCE-SITTER'

This nurse might say: *'The only way to behave in such uncertainty is to try mammography out and see, but keeping a "weather eye" on the programme monitoring and evaluation and keeping women aware of the uncertain position.'*

The advantages of Nurse Fence-Sitter's position are that she is being honest with the women thereby enhancing their autonomy and the women have a chance of being helped through the early diagnosis of breast cancer. The disadvantages are that the women she encounters may be confused and worried, they may not attend for breast screening and therefore have no opportunity of benefit. In addition, the programme is less likely to work due to poor attendance. There may also be a personal cost to the health promoter arising from her involvement with a programme that may not be working. The moral duties involved include veracity, respect for persons and non-maleficence.

Having looked more closely at the four Nurses views, the intriguing question is, who is behaving in the most ethical fashion? Is it Nurse Committed, Nurse Agin, Nurse Sidelines or Nurse Fence-Sitter?

Health education about mammography

Let us now leave this as food for thought for a moment and consider the question, how can we as health promoters educate women in this situation? Once again we shall examine how the various 'Nurses' above would approach this.

Nurse Committed might say to the women she is working with, *'Finding breast cancer early gives the best chance of cure, do go when invited.'*[1]

Alternatively, she might suggest, '*The benefit of being screened for breast cancer far outweighs any risk of harm, make sure you take advantage of the service.*'[2]

Nurse Agin might say in her work as a health promoter, '*Mammography does not offer women any benefit, I recommend you do not bother to go.*' In a stronger fashion she might say, '*Mammography is harmful, it should be stopped.*'

Nurse Sidelines might remain silent or say, '*I have no comment I cannot advise you about breast cancer screening.*'

Nurse Fence-Sitter might say, '*Mammography has possible benefits and drawbacks, it is very complex.*' She could then ask the woman what she wishes to know about mammography and drawing upon her communication skills she may try to convey some background facts in a manner appropriate to the individual woman. Nurse Fence-Sitter might draw upon some of the following information for this discussion.

- The woman's breast will need to be compressed to 4.5 cm (Forrest, 1990).
- 14 000 women will need to be screened to save one life (Rodgers, 1990).
- 142 000 women will be recalled with some false positives and some overdiagnosis (Rodgers, 1990).
- For every seven women found to have breast cancer, six will not live any longer as a result of early diagnosis (Rodgers, 1990).
- Some breast cancers will be missed at mammography (Rodgers, 1990; Skrabanek, 1989; Woods, 1991).
- Some cancers will develop in the three-year interval (Forrest, 1990).
- The cost of saving one life from screening is £80 000 (Rees, 1986).
- Treatment of breast cancer may include lumpectomy, mastectomy, radiotherapy, chemotherapy, hormone treatment.
- *Individual* benefit cannot be guaranteed (Skrabanek, 1990).

Having considered how the various 'Nurses' above would approach health education, it is interesting to ask, what are the strengths and weaknesses of these various ways of informing women?

Nurse Committed's information is clear, simple and persuasive. It is based on a professional's paternalistic judgement about what is of benefit to women and advises on that basis. Women are given clear simple guidance about their health and are spared the burden of assessing complicated evidence for themselves. At the same time, however, they receive little information about which to make their own judgements and remain dependent upon the health promoter. The women are therefore denied the opportunity to assess mammography for themselves and make a free choice on that basis. They may be harmed if the paternalistic judgement of the health promoter proves to have been incorrect or differs from the judgement that the women themselves would have made had they been given the opportunity.

Nurse Agin's information is clear, simple and persuasive. It too is based upon a professional's paternalistic judgement about what is of benefit to women and advises on that basis. The strengths and weaknesses of Nurse Agin's stance are very similar to those of Nurse Committed, as once again women are given clear, simple guidance about their health but little information upon which to make their own judgements.

Nurse Sidelines' information is straightforward and non-committal, it provides little information and does not advise. Women are given an honest response by the professional but receive no guidance about their health and no information about which to make their own judgements. This approach might be harmful if adopted by all health promoters.

Nurse Fence-Sitter's information depends to some extent upon her communication skills and her ability to respond to and convey a message appropriate to the individual women whose health she is concerned to promote. The information at her disposal is detailed, somewhat complicated and non-committal. Attempting to share this knowledge is based upon a belief in the need to respect a person's autonomy through informed consent. The women are given no advice and may be confused or alarmed, in addition they may be less likely to attend for breast screening. The women do, however, have a lot of information about which to make their own judgements. In addition, the health promoter has been honest with the women.

Which then is the most ethically sound approach in health promotion? Is the paternalism of Nurse Committed and Nurse Agin most appropriate, the 'neutrality' of Nurse Sidelines or the respect for autonomy through informed consent of Nurse Fence-Sitter?

The answer to this question is complex, it is worth considering some other questions which might help us as we think about our own view. In health promotion we are concerned with encouraging people to work with us as partners in safeguarding their health, enhancing and regaining control over their health. Two interesting questions are therefore, which of these approaches allows the woman to *participate* in her own health to the greatest degree? Which of these approaches *enables* the woman to increase control over her health? In addition, we might note that we accept both paternalistic judgements and those respecting autonomy through informed consent in caring for *patients*. Does the fact that *healthy people* are involved in breast cancer screening make any difference? What if we view women attending for mammography screening as *research subjects* how might this influence our health education as either paternalistic or respecting autonomy through informed consent? What if we view the women as *potential patients*, does this make any difference to health education? Does the question of whether the duty of the nurse is to the *individual* before her or to *society* as a whole have any relevance?

Conclusion

The ethical issues in mammography screening are paralleled in many other areas of health promotion. The evidence in this chapter suggests that nurses and other health promoters are placed in a difficult position in situations of such uncertainty. We need to debate the best way forward to be certain we are behaving in an ethical fashion.

This chapter has raised many questions and begun to answer only a few. These ideas are left as continuing food for thought and debate amongst nurses in their work as health promoters.

Acknowledgements

This chapter draws upon research being undertaken from Ph.D. studies. The research is being jointly supervised by Professor Jenifer Wilson-Barnett, Department of Nursing Studies, Kings College, University of London and Dr Alan Cribb, Lecturer in Ethics and Education, Centre for Educational Studies, Kings College, University of London.

Notes

1. The phrases used here are adapted from the Women's National Cancer Control Campaign (1989) leaflet entitled, 'Breast screening by mammography. Your questions answered', and the poster entitled, 'Have you heard about free breast screening?'
2. The phrases used here are adapted from the Women's National Cancer Control Campaign (1989) leaflet entitled, 'Breast screening by mammography. Your questions answered', and a Cancer Research Campaign (1991) leaflet entitled, 'Be breast aware'.

References

Department of Health and Social Security (1986). *Breast Cancer Screening.* Report to the Health Ministers of England, Wales, Scotland and Northern Ireland, by a working group chaired by Professor Sir Patrick Forrest. HMSO: London.

Department of Health (1992). *The Health of the Nation.* HMSO: London.

Forrest, P. (1990). *Breast Cancer: The Decision to Screen.* Nuffield Provincial Hospitals Trust: London.

Rees, G. (1986). Cost benefits of cancer services. *The Health Service Journal* (10 April), 490–1.

Rodgers, A. (1990). The UK breast cancer screening programme: an expensive mistake. *Journal of Public Health Medicine, 12,* 3–4, 197–204.

Schmidt, J. G. (1990). The epidemiology of mass breast cancer screening – a plea for a valid measure of benefit. *Journal of Clinical Epidemiology, 43,* 3, 215–25.

Skrabanek, P. (1989). Mass mammography. The time for reappraisal. *International Journal of Technology Assessment in Health Care, 5,* 423–30.

Tannahill, A. (1985). What is health promotion? *Health Education Journal, 44,* 167–8.

UK Trial of Early Detection of Breast Cancer Group (1988). First results on mortality reduction in the UK trial of early detection of breast cancer. *Lancet, ii,* 411–16.

Woods, M. (1991). Behind a screen. *Nursing Times* (27 November), *87,* 48.

7 Nursing as health promotion – a myth accepted?

Ursula Gallagher and Jerry Burden

Introduction

As nursing continues to strive for its definition and professional status it has looked to other disciplines for points of comparison. One area that has received much consideration is the interrelationship between nursing and health promotion. We chose this particular theme as we feel uncomfortable with what we see as an emerging trend within nursing theory. This trend is in turn exerting considerable pressure upon nursing, a pressure that seeks to equate nursing practice with health promotion activity. We are seeking to challenge and explore the ethical assumptions that underpin the claim that nursing practice is synonymous with health promotion.

At a time when nursing continues to struggle for its definition and professional status this equation will only lead to a confusion, to a myth.

We have therefore decided to try to dispel this myth. We believe it has developed through a misconception and confusion of the philosophical assumptions of each discipline which is in real danger of creating moral and epistemological problems for nursing and its practice.

This chapter will also explore the values that underlie how the two professions discuss the justification they have for the interventions. These are based on their understanding of philosophical concepts such as rights, duties and obligations and to what differing extent they consider that 'ought' means can. The chapter will present the argument that misconceptions have arisen because of a confusion of epistemology between the two professions. Using an analysis of the philosophical values of nursing and health promotion, the authors will analyse whether the words common to the language of both disciplines, e.g. autonomy, independence, actually share a common professional definition – it will be argued that they do not. Nursing has several unique elements to its practice and the authors will argue that

51

while health promotion may be an aspect of practice it does not subsume it.

Background

Two factors act as background to this chapter. The first is political and the second professional. The internal market now established within the NHS is demanding new responses from health care professionals. Purchasers are charged to secure health care as matches the needs of their local population. As this process matures their skills will be increasingly informed by the Health of the Nation, the Patients' Charter and the principles of WHO Health for All 2000. Consequently, it is clear that they will be ever more rigorous about the standards and quality of service than is currently being demanded. This means that nursing needs to be very explicit about what it has to offer. The current economic climate means that nursing skill mix is under great scrutiny and if nursing is seen to be encompassing health promotion, then they may soon find themselves obliged to provide such a service at the expense of bed-side care. Purchasers may not yet be able to quantify their standards about caring, but they can certainly stipulate what sort of health promotion interventions they believe the post-infarct patient will require.

The second factor is professional. Project 2000 and the Royal College of Nursing emphasise a double track approach to professional excellence; that of promoting health and caring for the sick. The fear is that one will become subsumed by the other; in this case that nursing will be unable to resist the pressure to adopt a greater health promotion role. In this scenario there is a danger that health promotion will become more valued than caring. In the light of the economic pressures on skill mix we have already mentioned this is a dangerous precedent. One which can only be exacerbated by the arrival of greater numbers of health care assistants. As they take on an increasing proportion of caring activity then just such a scenario might develop from an anticipated one to becoming a reality.

Our argument is simple. Nursing needs to re-evaluate its role in the context of the changes to the NHS. There is time to pause for breath from this headlong dash into health promotion and to reflect simply upon what nursing is trying to achieve.

Examining the assumptions

Health promotion

We begin by briefly examining the philosophical assumptions which underpin nursing and health promotion respectively. According to the WHO, 'Health is a broad, intercultural concept. It is the condition of physical, mental and social well-being and not merely the absence of disease or other abnormal conditions.' It describes an optimum ideal of health care which is beyond traditional conceptions predominant in the NHS delivery systems.

The WHO describes health promotion as 'the process of enabling people to increase control over and to improve their health'. Five principles underpin this description which helps incorporate a conceptual framework for health promotion;

1. Health promotion involves the population as a whole in the context of their lives rather than focusing on individuals at risk of disease.
2. Health promotion combines diverse but complementary methods.
3. Health promotion targets the determinants of health.
4. Health promotion is aimed at effective community participation.
5. Health promotion is basically a health and social activity and not a medical service.

Health is therefore viewed in a rather positive sense, concerned with the positive health and well-being rather than in the more negative mode of absence of disease or illness.

The initial conception was taken further in the Ottawa Charter for Health Promotion which reinforced the commitment to achieving equity in health, but went further in calling for the development of a specific health promotion policy which the charter outlined.

Health promotion policy combines diverse but complementary approaches including legislation, fiscal measures, taxation and organisational change. It is co-ordinated action that leads to health, income and social policies that foster greater equity. Joint action contributes to ensuring safer and healthier goods, healthier public services and cleaner, more enjoyable environments. (WHO, 1986)

Health promotion is not, therefore, theoretically concerned with individual behaviour as a major factor in current trends of ill health. Such emphasis on individual responsibility for health has raised issues of victim blaming for ill health and provided justifications for reductions in health care expenditure. Moreover, the health promotion approach seeks to redress the dominance of health care professionals within the medical environment. Not only is it concerned to criticise the influence of the medical model within health education (and perhaps health promotion), but also challenges the role health education professionals play in terms of their control and dictation of agendas. Such overt manipulation of communities, especially those who advocate or justify their actions in the name of 'empowerment', is simply unethical.

What these principles make clear is that health promotion is essentially an exercise in collective social activity. It is concerned with creating the context in which the enabling process can occur. Therefore, it has as its agenda such ideas as healthy public policy (seeking to place health in as many public policy agendas as possible); to influence social and economic policy and to advocate for an environment where the health choice is the easy choice for individuals. However, it is not in dispute that nursing has a role to play within the wider political area, that seeks real health change by addressing the underlying structural forces that influence society.

Nursing and caring

Nursing, we suggest, has caring firmly rooted in its belief system and practice. Brenner and Wrubel (1989) argue that, 'Caring is primary because it sets up the possibility of giving help and receiving help.' This establishes a relationship, an *individual* relationship between nurse and patient where care can be directly negotiated with the patient or family. It is this relationship based upon as assessment and evaluation of individual needs which sets nursing apart from other health care professionals. It is probably one of nursing's greatest strengths.

Brenner and Wrubel (1989) demonstrate the strength of this relationship when they state: 'This enabling condition of connection and concern is another way in which caring is primary. Caring (about someone or something) places the person in the situation in such a way that certain aspects show up as relevant.' By emphasising what is important to the individual, nursing is confronted by divergent and shifting perceptions of health. It is not for nurses to impose a preconceived idea of health on to patients. Nursing should not be concerned with handing out advice to people based on personal preference and anecdotal evidence. Nurses should not be engaged in offering people an optimal vision of health which they might not be able to achieve, nor may not even wish to. Instead nurses are in a unique position within the health care system as, via the nursing process, they have the opportunity effectively to assess an individual's own perception of what their health means to them. It is a chance to negotiate health goals and aims, to set targets which the individual and the nurse can work together to achieve. And it is only through this process of negotiation and assessment of individual need by skilled professionals that a truly therapeutic relationship can evolve.

The epistemological confusions

We can demonstrate this confusion further if we examine words, which on the surface appear common to the language of both professions, but in fact do not have a shared definition of interpretation. Both health promotion and nursing, as we have noted, lay claim to an empowerment function both as a process, which informs their practice, and as a hoped for outcome of the interventions. However, interventions in the name of enablement require permission from the people involved and it is to the area of consent that we now turn.

We suggest that the important differences between nursing and health promotion conceptions of enablement are influenced by divergent positions on health. Within health promotion, empowerment is more often a smoke screen for a more passing assumption. Health promotion activity, whether in the form of life skills training of health education through to the intended outcome of individuals hopefully making healthy choices, is underpinned by the assumption that there is a need for change, a need to alter health behaviour and lifestyle in favour of what health promoters consider to be more appropriate. It is also underpinned by the belief that health promotion provides the best indicator of how that change might be achieved.

Empowerment theories remain the most problematic within either health education or health promotion. Yet they may hold the key to achieving the kind of balance Baric (1985) talks about, while at the same time strengthening the kind of community action essential to achieve Health for All 2000. Tones *et al.* (1990) appears to make this point when he argues for the centrality of empowerment models within health education. He claims that self-empowerment has a crucial facilitating function in relation to preventive and radical (social) models of health education. This function is designed to improve individuals or the community's ability to make informed choices and decisions by enhancing concepts of self-esteem and self-confidence. The crux of the theory is that such individual or community participation is not true participation in programmes handed down from experts but rather involves the community 'deciding about their needs and taking over responsibility for activities aimed at meeting those needs'. It is only when equity begins at the bottom that it can ever be realised at the top.

However, this need for change is made on behalf of the population. There is no contract, either existing or pending, which could legitimise such an intervention. There is no discussion as to the nature of the intervention or whether change is actually desired. In short, there is no consent; hence the charge of paternalism.

In contrast, nursing cannot and must not lay itself open to such a criticism. Historically, nursing has intervened to do for the patient what they would otherwise do for themselves were they not ill. Traditional methods of organising care have taken this benevolent assumption to its logical conclusion, i.e. task allocation and routining of ward activity, but this is now changing. As primary nursing becomes more prevalent, as its philosophy and practice become more readily acceptable, so nursing has started to re-evaluate how it legitimises its practice.

In our opinion the enabling process within nursing practice is conditioned by the principles of caring outlined previously. There is no fixed process, nor are there fixed outcomes. Nursing must accept the individual as seen and then, and only then can it seek to offer skills and advice. This principle of acceptance is directly compatible with negotiation about

- what sort of intervention is actually required;
- who should actually perform this activity.

Nursing therefore seeks the consent of the people it cares for. It does not blithely assume that it has the right to intervene on their behalf. More importantly, it does not often instil a sense that change is not only necessary but not to do so is also wrong.

Within this relationship there are no mass statistical targets to be achieved. There is no political agenda to be satisfied. There is simply the satisfaction of being involved in a freely negotiated enabling process. We agree with Tones *et al.* (1990) that nursing has a role to play within this process, but it is in danger of losing sight of this particular strength if the emphasis continues to shift away from accepting and caring for individuals.

Stemming from this line of argument are further ethical and epistemological problems. It is simply not ethical to encourage people that they ought to do something if they do not have the capacity to do so. For example, encouraging people to eat healthier foods is unethical if the healthier choice is not available either in local shops or at a price that is affordable. Furthermore, it is unjustified to attempt to promote any activity which is not a negotiated outcome. It is ludicrous to tell people that they ought to stop smoking without actually asking them whether or not it is something they wish to do. Thus if health promotion wishes to work with the maxim 'ought means can', then it is important that it is able to work both on the demand and supply side of the health equilibrium.

Health promotion therefore needs to examine closely its role within these two areas. On the demand side, it can and does campaign for people to choose the healthier option in their diet and lifestyle. Health promotion maintains an advocacy role on behalf of the public in an attempt to create a demand for a wider choice for consumers which would include healthier products. The problem for health promotion is that it cannot sustain that role unless it is also able to influence the supply side as well. Can it persuade government to introduce policies which regulate misleading advertisements and health information?

Can it influence manufacturers and retailers to adjust their product range and pricing strategy in the direction of wider health promotion aims?

In turn, this reflects the epistemological problems within health promotion. These surround issues of data and data collection and whether clinical epidemiology is the correct method of collecting and collating the information necessary to be able to justify health promotion interventions. As purchasing authorities are now more concerned with assessing local health needs as a base for service provision, so what role will there be for target setting imposed from the WHO? Who sets these targets? Are they negotiated or imposed? Why are they set at these levels? These are questions that require careful answers because if health promotion is unable to convince people that its knowledge base is sufficient to justify its interventions, then how will it refute the claim that it treats people as object rather than subject? Such problems cannot help but shape the nature of health promotion interventions.

Undoubtedly, health promotion has a role to play and something unique and positive to offer the health of the UK. We agree that the environment is a central issue. We applaud health promoters' determination to tackle health inequalities and health equity. It is simply that we feel that some of its weaknesses and problems also need to be explored and exposed before nursing begins to try to make use of it. Furthermore, we believe nursing can and should avoid the pitfalls outlined above. Research has suggested that nurses are not terribly good at listening, at communicating information or even, as we suggest, negotiation.

Nursing has worked hard at developing its own knowledge base to inform its practice and the way it should organise itself to deliver care. We feel that just as nursing is finally coming to terms with the concept of caring, with the idea of putting patients before routines, that to embrace a whole new concept and to use it as a legitimising tool for nursing practice is simply misguided.

Conclusion

What is needed is essentially a breathing space for an intellectual time out. Nursing needs to take a long look at health promotion and understand the theoretical considerations that underpin its practice, its strengths and weaknesses, the relevant areas for nursing to explore and the relationship between nursing practice and health promotion.

We do not believe that enough time or effort has been given over to this exercise. The result has been the sort of philosophical and ethical confusion we have described above.

We strongly believe that there is a real danger that in the future nursing activity could well restrict itself to the health promotion role only. This would not be the route to professional excellence. In fact it would merely serve to deskill what is an informed and intelligent profession. It is only when we recognise this danger that nursing will be in a position to explore what health promotion has to offer nursing – but more importantly, what nursing has to offer health promotion.

References

Baric, L. (1985). The meaning of words: health promotion. *Journal of the Institute of Health Education, 23,* 10–15.

Brenner, P. and Wrubel, J. (1989). *The primacy of caring: Stress and Coping in Health and Illness.* Addison-Wesley Publishing Co., New York.

Tones, K., Tilford, S. and Robinson, Y. (1990). *Health Education: Effectiveness and Efficiency.* Chapman & Hall: London, Chapter 1.

World Health Organization (1986). Ottowa Charter for Health Promotion. An International Conference on Health Promotion (17–21 November). WHO Regional Office for Europe: Copenhagen.

Health Promotion in Practice

This section examines the role of nurses and other staff as health promotion agents with those who are sick and vulnerable. Resulting from a major study at King's College, London, a survey of acute hospitals in England demonstrates that despite some awareness that a new shift in priorities is needed, little real progress has been made. Even more worrying are the findings from a qualitative study by Meyer (see Chapter 11) in which the barriers erected by staff to patients' and family participation are outlined and interpreted. The evidence from chapters on community staff points to their potential as promoters of health, the various effects of health visitors' communication with clients and the practice nurses' motivation to become more pro-active through education.

Even though general findings may not be overwhelmingly positive or impressive, greater staff understanding and apparent willingness to be involved in health promoting activities may lead to more initiatives and more genuine attitudes. Examples of transcripts and opportunities outlined in some of these chapters may help to sensitise others to their own style of communication and give meaning to the term 'health promotion' in acute care settings. Community staff may also be helped to identify ways in which they can help other staff, and of course themselves, to accept the role of supporting troubled families which has been generally neglected.

8 Factors influencing nurses' health education and health promotion practice in acute ward areas

Jenifer Wilson-Barnett and Sue Latter

Introduction

This chapter outlines selected findings from a two-year Department of Health funded research project entitled 'Health Education and Health Promotion in Nursing: A Study of Practice in Acute Areas'. The overall aims of the study were: (i) to describe the extent to which health education and health promotion had become integrated into nurses' practice in acute care settings and (ii) to identify the facilitative and inhibitory factors involved. The study comprised three stages of data collection and utilised a multimethod approach which is described more fully below. The focus of this chapter concerns the factors which were identified as influential in the development of health education and health promotion at ward level. Findings from a survey of ward sisters and from ward-based case studies are presented and discussed.

Literature

Despite the recent recommendations urging all nurses to develop their health education and health promotion role (e.g. Department of Health, 1989; Royal College of Nursing, 1989), there has been relatively little research in this area, particularly in relation to nurses working in hospital settings. To date, research has focused on nursing and medical staff working in the community (e.g. Catford and Nutbeam, 1983; Sanders *et al.*, 1986; Hinds *et al.*, 1987) and the literature on health education and health promotion in acute sector nursing is predominantly prescriptive or confined to small-scale research studies evaluating the impact of health education initiatives.

However, two recent studies which did derive data from hospital settings suggest that currently nurses' health education and health promotion practice is limited. Johnston's (1988) single site study involved interviews with fifty randomly selected patients on general surgical wards and revealed a singular lack of advice given by nursing and medical staff in relation to lifestyles. Gott and O'Brien's work in 1990 examined nurses' perceptions of their health education role and practice and observation of their performance in a variety of settings. They found that nurses in hospital settings in particular 'remained locked into routinized systems and practices' and that ideas of partnership and participation had not yet found their way on to nurses' agendas.

These findings suggest that nurses' performance falls short of the recommendations referred to earlier. It would therefore seem important to identify the factors which either facilitate or inhibit this aspect of hospital nurses' practice. A review of the relevant literature indicates that a number of potentially important variables emerge. Lack of time has frequently been cited as a factor inhibiting nurses' ability to put health education into practice (Winslow, 1976; Murdaugh, 1980; Ruzicki, 1987; Tilley et al., 1987; Wilson-Barnett, 1988; Dudley, 1990) and this has often been associated with a heavy workload and inadequate staffing levels (e.g. Coxon, 1986; Honan et al., 1988). Nurses' lack of knowledge is also frequently suggested as a difficulty (Elkind, 1982; Schuster and Jones, 1982; Gleit and Graham, 1985). Research-based evidence also points to this conclusion: Faulkner and Ward's (1983) study of attitudes of hospital nurses towards health education and smoking revealed that the nurses had a poor knowledge base about smoking which inhibited their willingness and ability to act as health educators. Similarly, Macleod Clark et al.'s (1985) research found a lack of knowledge existed in relation tó the physiological effects of smoking and smoking cessation advice. Other potentially important factors that have been suggested include the role of the ward sister (Syred, 1981), the self-sentiment of the nurses themselves (Clarke, 1991; Vaughan, 1991) including self-knowledge and empowerment, and the continuity afforded by the system of organising nursing care (Murdaugh, 1980; Tilley et al., 1987). However, many of these assertions are unsubstantiated by research or are based on small-scale surveys of nurses' perceptions, and thus the importance of research into this largely unexplored area becomes clear. The study described below attempts to address this gap in the research literature at a time when health education and health promotion are assuming increasing importance in nursing.

Methods

(1) Semi-structured interviews were conducted with 132 ward sisters in nine District Health Authorities throughout England. The sample was selected on the basis of responses to a national postal survey which formed the first stage of the project (see Latter *et al.*, 1992). Respondents were asked to describe the extent to which health education and health promotion had become integrated into practice on their respective wards and to identify the influential factors involved.

(2) Data were collected on a subsample of six case study wards involving self-administered questionnaires (n = 62), two hour periods of non-participant observation (n = 67), tape recordings of significant incidents (n = 48) and field notes made by the researchers. The wards were selected from the ward sister interview sample in an attempt to identify potential models of good practice. Thus, key criteria for selection were the range of health education and health promotion activities described and the ward sister's level of understanding of the concepts and the issues involved in implementing them.

Data from both stages were analysed using both quantitative and qualitative approaches.

Results

Ward sister interviews

Ward sisters' responses to the question of whether or not nurses were engaged in health education and health promotion activities are shown in *Figure 8.1*. Further analysis of the types of activities that nurses were perceived to be involved in revealed a focus on patient education and information-giving (n = 104 and 60 respectively). Encouraging patient and relative participation in care were less frequently identified by respondents as being carried out by nurses (n = 13 and 27 respectively). This finding is closely linked to the way in which ward sisters interpreted the terms health education and health promotion. That is, their perceptions were characterised by an illness-oriented focus, largely derived from a medical model of care and lacked recognition of the major concepts inherent in the newer paradigms of health education and health promotion such as collaboration, participation and empowerment.

The ward sisters also identified a range of factors which were considered either to inhibit or to facilitate nurses' ability to put health education and health promotion into practice on their wards. Results

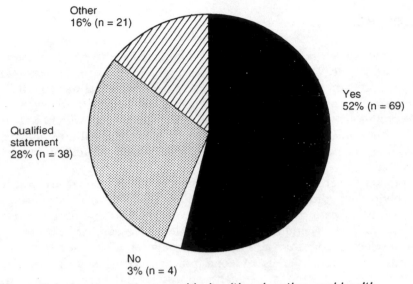

Figure 8.1 *Are nurses engaged in health education and health promotion? . . . Ward sisters' responses*

are shown in *Tables 8.1* and *8.2*. Lack of time was the most frequently identified difficulty and this was commonly associated with such hindrances and inadequate staffing, heavy workload, other nursing care priorities and the increasingly short length of patient admissions. The prevalence with which lack of time was cited is inextricably linked to respondents' understandings of the concepts. That is, whether health education and health promotion are viewed as isolated activities to be added on to care if there is time, or whether they are seen as integral to all care and thus able to be incorporated into a nurse's approach to any care activity.

Patient factors were felt to exert an inhibitory influence by 67 per cent (n = 88) of the sample. This referred to such ideas as the acuity of the patient's illness or their willingness to listen to advice and/or alter their behaviour. Factors pertaining to nurses were also considered problematic by 41 per cent (n = 54) of respondents and included such comments as nurses' motivation to implement health education activities and the fact that they were often unhealthy role models.

Table 8.2 shows that overall fewer numbers of respondents identified current or potential facilitative influences and many of those cited were the opposite of their counterpart inhibitory influence. Those most frequently identified concerned the provision of sufficient health education and promotion resources such as leaflets and posters (n = 72, 54 per cent). Just over a third of respondents (n = 34, 46 per cent) identified organising care via a system of primary or team nursing as a

Table 8.1 *Factors inhibiting health education and health promotion practice cited by ward sisters (n = 132)*

Factors identified by ward sisters	No. of ward sisters	%
Lack of time	107	81
Patient factors	88	67
Lack of knowledge/skill	70	53
Nurse factors	54	41
Patients' length of stay	46	35
Inadequate staffing	44	33
Priorities	40	30
Medical staff	28	21
Workload	26	20
Interference with patients' freedom to choose/quality of life	22	17

Table 8.2 *Factors facilitating health education and health promotion practice spontaneously cited by ward sisters (n = 132)*

Factors identified by sisters	Current facilitating factors		Potential facilitating factors		Total	
	n	%	n	%	n	%
Health education/ promotion resources	53	40	19	14	72	54
Nurse factors	43	32	1	1	44	33
Organisation of care	40	30	6	4	46	34
Patient factors	37	28	0	0	37	28
Shared philosophy of care	25	19	4	3	29	22
Nurses' knowledge	21	16	1	1	22	17
More time	18	13	13	10	31	23
Staff development and training	18	13	7	5	25	18
Good multidisciplinary liaison	13	10	2	2	15	12

beneficial influence, and this was substantiated by findings from the case study wards.

Smaller numbers of respondents identified broader, more philo-sophical influences such as nurses' philosophical approach to care and a supportive ward climate as being important. These respondents tended to have a more comprehensive understanding of the concepts and of the issues involved in implementing them.

The collection of data on the case study wards enabled the significance in reality of these perceived influences on practice to be determined and the findings are presented below.

Case study wards

Analysis of data collected from the six case study wards revealed a range in the extent to which health education and health promotion had become integrated into nurses' practice. The results indicated that wards could best be depicted according to their place on a continuum of practice, as shown in *Figure 8.2.*

Thus the wards ranged from one ward on which there was an absence of any health education and promotion practice to two wards where practice could be considered to be at an advanced level. On the former, the data revealed that nurses were operating with a predominantly medical model of care with a physical task orientation and attempts made by patients to participate in care were blocked by nurses. In contrast, on wards 3 and 4 nurses' practice was characterised by information giving and explanation in most interventions and patient participation in events such as bedside handover. However, these wards fell short of what was considered a comprehensive level of

Absent	Minimal	Emerging	Advanced	Comprehensive
Ward 5	Ward 2	Wards 1 and 6	Wards 3 and 4	
Lack of info-giving	Some info-giving	Preparatory info-giving	Health promoting approach	
Participation blocked		Routine opportunity of education	Explanation in most interventions	
Physical task oriented		at discharge (top down)	Bedside handovers with patients participating	
			Little healthy lifestyle advice	
			Missed opportunities patient and relative participation	

Figure 8.2 *Levels of health education/health promotion practice*

practice in that there was little evidence of health lifestyle advice being offered to patients and opportunities for patient and relative participation in care were sometimes missed.

Analysis of questionnaire data and of the researchers' field notes, as well as some cross-case comparison, enabled a number of key influences on nurses' practice to be identified and these are shown in *Figure 8.3*.

Philosophical approach to care

Importantly, data on the reality of nurses' practice showed that the broader, more philosophical influences identified by a small number of

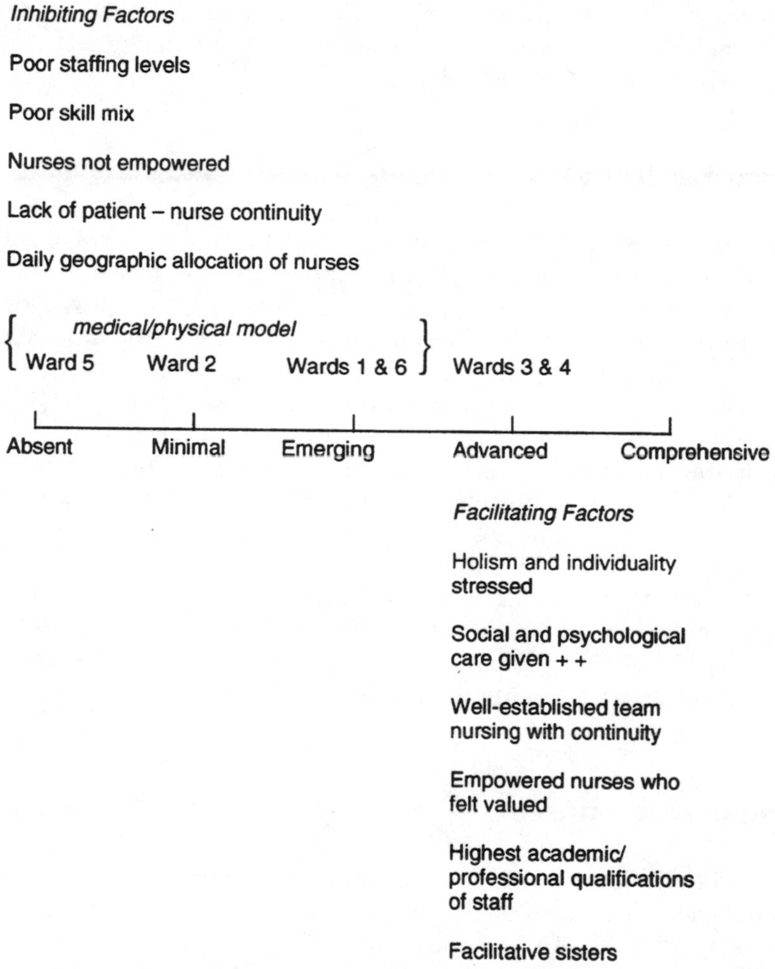

Inhibiting Factors

Poor staffing levels

Poor skill mix

Nurses not empowered

Lack of patient – nurse continuity

Daily geographic allocation of nurses

{ *medical/physical model*
Ward 5   Ward 2   Wards 1 & 6 } Wards 3 & 4

Absent   Minimal   Emerging   Advanced   Comprehensive

Facilitating Factors

Holism and individuality stressed

Social and psychological care given + +

Well-established team nursing with continuity

Empowered nurses who felt valued

Highest academic/ professional qualifications of staff

Facilitative sisters

Figure 8.3 *Levels of health education/health promotion practice*

respondents were highly significant in influencing nurses' ability to integrate health education and health promotion into ward-based practice. Data from wards on which health education and health promotion were considered to be at an 'advanced' level of integration by the research team indicated that a number of factors provided the necessary infrastructure for this development. First, the underlying philosophical approach to care conducive to health education and health promotion is one which embraces holism and individuality such that the patient's psychological and social well-being is addressed, together with an approach to the patient characterised by respect and nurse–patient collaboration and equality. Conversely, the wards on which least development had occurred were operating with an underlying medical model of care, which militates against nurses' involvement in health education and health promotion work with patients. On these wards, practice was characterised by an emphasis on the completion of physical care tasks as well as a 'top down' approach to any advice or information giving.

Organization of care

Case study ward data also confirmed the facilitative influences of team or primary nursing: this was seen to offer continuity of care, individual responsibility and autonomy for nurse practitioners, thus providing a base from which trusting and supportive nurse–patient relationships could develop and health education and health promotion flourish. Conversely, on wards with discontinuous and anonymous individual nurse–patient allocation, health education and health promotion were poorly developed due to the fragmentary nature of care giving and practitioners' lack of individual responsibility for patients' care. The ability to implement an effective system of team or primary nursing was also found to be dependent on adequate numbers of appropriately skilled staff. Thus, staffing levels and skill mix are also influential in nurses' ability to put health education and health promotion into practice, although this may not always be directly related to the availability of time for these activities *per se*, as nurses' perceptions would suggest.

Empowered nurses

Secondly, the data revealed that the ward climate needs to be such that nurses feel valued, supported, autonomous and empowered members of the ward team. This appeared to facilitate health education and health promotion via increasing morale and enabling nurses to support and empower their patients rather than maintain traditional role distinctions and the unequal balance of power inherent in these. This support and empowerment of nurses was closely associated with a democratic management style from the ward sister such that each nurse was individually responsible for decisions regarding care and whose opinion was respected and listened to. Thus, the facilitative influence of primary or team nursing is again highlighted, it being characterised by a flattened ward hierarchy and devolved decision-making. Conversely, on wards where the traditional hierarchy remained intact, nurses were disempowered and their opinions often not sought or respected, leading to low morale and a need to retain power and control over their patients. As a consequence, health education and health promotion were poorly developed or absent on these wards.

The ward sister

Finally, data from these case study wards also revealed the crucial significance of the ward sister in facilitating or inhibiting nurses' health education and health promotion practice. The foregoing discussion makes clear her pivotal role in instigating the necessary infrastructure, that is, encouraging a certain philosophical approach to care, developing team or primary nursing, and offering support and empowerment to individual nurses through a democratic style of management. The ward sister's influence as a role model and in establishing a ward climate in which learning and knowledge acquisition were regarded as important were also found to be facilitative influences on the wards where most progress in terms of health education and health promotion practice had been made. In addition, the two wards on which practice was most advanced were staffed by ward sisters and nursing staff who were amongst those who had obtained the highest academic and professional qualifications of the sample.

Conclusion

Findings from interviews with ward sisters and from a number of case study wards indicate that there is a range in the extent to which health education and health promotion are both perceived and observed to have become a feature of nurses' practice in acute ward settings. The findings suggest that currently nurses are not fulfilling their potential and this therefore highlights the need to examine the factors which both facilitate and inhibit this aspect of their role in order to guide future policy and practice. This research-based chapter has outlined a number of important influences identified by both ward sisters and observation of the reality of nurses' practice. Findings from the interviews with ward sisters indicate that the most commonly identified influences are inextricably related to these nurses' understandings of what the concepts of health education and health promotion represent (which forms the basis of chapter 9 in this book). The influential factors identified by the ward sisters also bear a close resemblance to those previously identified in the literature, with lack of time and knowledge featuring prominently. In contrast, findings from the case study wards revealed a number of more global, structural influences at work such as nurses' philosophical approach to care and the way in which care is organised and allocated on a day to day basis. Whilst the factors identified by the ward sisters are not regarded as unimportant, and may be necessary adjuncts to successful health education and promotion practice, these may be addressed by an increased understanding of what the concepts represent via educational input. The implications of the findings from the case study wards are that nurses should continue to strive for care that is individualised and holistically based and delivered via a system of organisation of care that offers continuity, autonomy, responsibility, and maximises the potential for empowerment of nurses. The ward sister is instrumental in implementing this necessary infrastructure and future efforts to integrate health education and health promotion into acute ward nurses' practice may best be channelled through her, together with other necessary and supportive changes at ward and organisational level.

References

Catford, J. C. and Nutbeam, D. (1983). Promoting health, preventing disease: what should the NHS be doing now? *Health Educational Journal, 42*, 1, 7–12.

Clarke, A. C. (1991). Nurses as role models and health educators. *Journal of Advanced Nursing, 16*, 1178–84.

Coxon, J. (1986). Health education: A learning dilemma. *Senior nurse, 5*, 1, 22–4.

Department of Health (1989). *A Strategy for Nursing.* A report of the Steering Committee. Department of Health Nursing Division: London.

Dudley, A. (1990). *Educating Patients in Hospital; Nurses' Decision Making Processes.* Unpublished study undertaken as part of the Burford Research in Clinical Nursing Course, 1989–90.

Elkind, A. K. (1982). Nurses views about cancer. *Journal of Advanced Nursing, 7*, 43–50.

Faulkner, A. and Ward, L. (1983). Nurses as health educators in relation to smoking. *Nursing Times, 79*, 8, 47–8.

Gleitt, C. J. and Graham, B. A. (1985). Reading materials used in the preparation of nurses for the teaching role. *Patient Education and Counselling, 6*, 1, 25–8.

Gott, M. and O'Brien, M. (1990). *The Role of the Nurse in Health Promotion: Policies, Perspectives, and Practice.* Report of a 2-year project funded by the Department of Health, London.

Hinds, P. S. and Young, K. J. (1987). A triangulation of methods and paradigms to study nurse given wellness-care. *Nursing Research, 36,* 3, 195–8.

Honan, S., Krsnak, G., Petersen, D. and Torkelson, R. (1988). The nurse as patient educator: perceived responsibilities and factors enhancing role development. *Journal of Continuing Education in Nursing, 19,* 1, 33–7.

Johnston, I. (1988). *A Study of the Promotion of Healthy Lifestyles by Hospital Based Staff.* Unpublished M.Sc. thesis, University of Birmingham.

Latter, S., Macleod Clark, J., Wilson-Barnett, J. and Maben, J. (1992). Health education in nursing: perceptions of practice in acute settings. *Journal of Advanced Nursing, 17,* 1, 164–72.

Macleod Clark, J., Elliott, K., Haverty, S. and Kendall, S. (1985). *Helping Patients and Clients to Stop Smoking – the Nurse's Role.* Department of Nursing Studies, King's College London.

Murdaugh, C. (1980). Effects of nurses' knowledge of teaching – learning principles on knowledge of coronary care unit patients. *Heart and Lung, 9,* 6, 1073–8.

RCN (1989). *Into the Nineties: Promoting Professional Excellence.* Royal College of Nursing: London.

Ruzicki, D. A. (1987). Staff involvement in patient teaching: making it happen. *Patient Education and Counselling, 10,* 83–9.

Sanders, D. J., Stone, V., Fowler, G. and Marzillier, J. (1986). Practice nurses and anti-smoking education. *British Medical Journal, 292,* 381–4.

Schuster, P. and Jones, S. (1982). Preparing the patient for a barium enema: a comparison of nurse and patient opinions. *Journal of Advanced Nursing, 7,* 523–7.

Syred, M. E. J. (1981). The abdication of the role of health education by hospital nurses. *Journal of Advanced Nursing, 6,* 27–33.

Tilley, J. D., Gregor, F. M. and Thiessen, V. (1987). The nurses role in patient education: incongruent perceptions among patients and nurses. *Journal of Advanced Nursing, 12,* 3, 291–301.

Vaughan, B. (1991). *Nursing as Therapy.* Ed. McMahon, R. and Pearson, A. Chapman & Hall, London.

Wilson-Barnett, J. (1988). Patient teaching or patient counselling? *Journal of Advanced Nursing, 13,* 215–22.

Winslow, E. H. (1976). The role of the nurse in patient education. *Nursing Clinics of North America, 11,* 2, 213–22.

9 Health education and health promotion in acute ward settings: nurses' perceptions and practice

Sue Latter

Introduction

This chapter describes one aspect of the results of a Department of Health funded research project examining nurses' health education and health promotion practice in acute ward settings. The data presented focus on ward-based nurses' interpretations of the concepts of health education and health promotion and their role in this, and the relationship between these perceptions and nurses' health education and health promotion practice in these settings.

Background

Against a backdrop of recent social, economic and demographic trends and changes in patterns of morbidity and mortality, health education and the promotion of health have assumed increasing importance in today's society. Simultaneously, the central position of nurses as educators and promoters of health has been recognised and calls have been made for them to adopt a leadership role in this respect. Accordingly, the nursing profession's statutory bodies and professional organisations have emphasised the importance of the nurse's role in health education and health promotion. For example, in its *A Strategy for Nursing*, the Department of Health (1989: 34) recommends that one target for practice is that: 'Health education and health promotion should be a recognized part of health care; all practitioners should develop skills in, and use every opportunity for, health promotion.' Whilst health education and health promotion have traditionally been regarded as the responsibility of nurses' working in primary health care settings, more recently the opportunities afforded to hospital-based nurses have also been recognised (e.g. RCN, 1989).

However, little attempt has been made in the nursing literature to clarify what is meant by 'health education' or 'health promotion' and hospital nurses' role in this. Rather, the recommendations that have been made assume a common understanding of these terms and there is therefore no attempt to clarify the hospital-based nurse's role in health education and health promotion. This presumed unanimity stands in direct contrast to the debate that has been raging in the health education and health promotion literature during the past two decades over the meaning ascribed to these concepts. The lack of agreement is such that Saunders (1988) was prompted to remark that the definition depends on who you ask. Gott and O'Brien (1990) add that meaning given to these concepts is inseparable from the agenda of the defining parties.

Given this lack of consensus, the minimal exploration of this issue in the nursing literature and in the absence of any directive from statutory or professional bodies, nurses' own individual interpretation of the concepts of health education and health promotion could be expected to exert a significant influence on their practice. That is, nurses' understanding of these terms is likely to act as a conceptual framework from which certain activities and approaches to health education and health promotion are derived and operationalised in practice. It therefore follows that a close relationship between nurses' perceptions and their practice may be expected to exist.

Literature review

In spite of the potential significance of this area, there has been little research which focuses specifically on hospital nurses' perceptions and practice of health education and health promotion. The only available research on practitioners' interpretation of these concepts is almost exclusively derived from those working in community settings and focuses on health care professionals other than nurses (e.g. Collins, 1984; Nutbeam, 1984; Rawson and Grigg, 1988). One study which did focus on nurses was conducted by Gott and O'Brien (1990). Semi-structured interviews and non-participant observation techniques were used to derive data from nurses working in a variety of settings to investigate . . . 'how the perceptions and practices of nurses connected with the major principles of health promotion philosophy as it is currently understood'. The authors concluded that for nurses in their study, health promotion corresponded to an attempt to persuade, cajole or otherwise influence individuals to alter their lifestyles. Gott and O'Brien concluded that in spite of recognising the existence and potential impact of wider variables in the economy, government and society, great emphasis was placed on the risk factors of smoking, drinking, stress, dietary and exercise habits of individuals and 'there was little evidence that the agenda of the patients and clients – even less of the public at large – had found its way into nursing's understanding of the potential re-orientation that health promotion principles offer'. However, the concepts and ideologies held by hospital nurses specifically remain unclear as, deliberately, the authors did not distinguish between groups of nurses working in community, school, occupational health and hospital settings. In addition, the above study did not set out explicitly to address the relationship between nurses' perceptions and their practice: rather, the aim was to examine the relationships between the roles played by nurses and the *contexts* in which those roles are undertaken.

The research study presented below therefore attempted to redress this potentially significant gap in the research literature at a time when health education and health promotion are assuming increasing importance to hospital-based nurses.

Methods

Data were collected in two principal stages, on both nurses' perceptions and observation of the reality of nurses' practice:

- Semi-structured interviews were conducted with a sample of 132 ward sisters and charge nurses on acute wards in nine District Health Authorities throughout England. The sample was selected on the basis of a preceding national survey of senior nurse managers (see Latter *et al.*, 1992). These interviews began with an open-ended question requiring the ward sister or charge nurse to clarify what the terms 'health education' and 'health promotion' meant to them and to describe any perceived distinction between the two.
- Data were subsequently collected on a subsample of six case study wards. Methods employed involved self-administered questionnaires to all ward-based staff (n = 62); non-participant focused observation of nurses' practice; tape recordings of nurse–patient interactions (n = 48), and field notes made by the researchers.

Results

Interpretation of the concepts of health education and health promotion

In general, ward sisters' responses were characterised by some degree of hesitancy and confusion. Qualitative analysis of the data revealed that the major categories that emerged did not relate specifically or consistently to either 'health education' or 'health promotion' and so the findings are presented without distinguishing between the two concepts. The ward sisters' understandings of the concepts were found to be characterised by a number of features.

First, there was an emphasis on preventing, or coping with illness as opposed to the promotion of positive health. Many comments reflected this illness orientation. The following are a sample:

> If I talk about health education, I tend to be talking about people who are ill, who need to understand their illness, or either adapt their lifestyle or live within their limitations.

> I suppose . . . most of the patients have ongoing illnesses really, like diabetes and heart failure, and so its aiming to help them to come to some acceptance of that, of their ongoing conditions.

This emphasis on helping patients to cope with already existing illness is similar to the idea of tertiary prevention as opposed to health education aimed at primary or secondary prevention. In addition, responses were characterised by a focus on physical health and disease – very few mentioned mental or social components of health.

Second, health education and health promotion were felt to consist of information and advice giving, predominantly about patients' lifestyles. In particular, the content of this lifestyle advice was generally perceived to revolve around the issues of diet and smoking, as the following comments illustrate:

> Health promotion means saying to the patients before they go home about smoking, eating a healthy diet and anti-stress techniques.

> Health education . . . I see it as closely linked to health promotion . . . we try to discourage people from smoking and make them aware of losing weight if they need to lose weight, and eating healthily.

In this sense, nurses' perceptions were similar to those of nurses in Gott and O'Brien's (1990) study. Responses also demonstrated a lack of recognition of the wider social, economic and political determinants of health and therefore clearly reflected on an individualistic, reductionist approach to health education and health promotion.

Third, respondents saw health promotion and their role in this as revolving around activities at the one–one, nurse–patient level. This is obviously related to the above finding that health promotion consists largely of individual lifestyle counselling. There was an emphasis on advising, educating and informing individual patients as opposed to a recognition that health promotion can involve alternative ways of working, such as intersectoral planning, action on issues affecting health, and involvement in planning and implementing health promoting policy such as smoke-free hospitals and healthy menu options for patients. The following responses reflect this interpretation:

> Health education suggests to me someone who is in need of being taught specific things.

> Health education conjures ideas about advising, sharing information with individuals in relation to healthy options and disease processes.

> Health promotion is a system of giving health information to individual patients – it's information giving.

These ward sisters' responses revealed a lack of recognition that the education process should be two-way and participatory, in keeping with current health promotion philosophy.

Finally, and linked to all of the above findings, ward sisters' responses to the question on their understandings of health education and health promotion were lacking in any mention of concepts currently believed to be central to health education and health promotion. Thus, none of the ward sisters referred to such concepts as collaboration, equity, participation and empowerment.

These findings clearly have implications for the types of activities that are being developed in the name of health education and health promotion in acute ward settings. The data collected from six case study wards allowed exploration of the reality of nurses' practice and the main findings are summarised below.

Nurses' health education and health promotion practice

Analysis of the data collected indicated that although there was a *range* in the quantity and quality of nurses' practice, certain conclusions could be drawn which very closely mirrored respondents' perceptions of what health education and health promotion represent and their role in this.

First, information and advice giving about coping with illness seemed to represent the predominant way in which nurses were developing their health promotion role. This was a feature of practice on most of the case study wards. For example patients on a surgical ward were offered preparatory advice about surgery and the post-operative period. Much of this information could be said to be of a tertiary preventive nature – very little evidence was collected of nurses' involvement in activities aimed at the promotion of positive health or with a primary prevention focus. Quite clearly, nurses' perceptions and their practice are similar in this respect.

In addition, case study ward data showed that nurses' health promotion work was focused exclusively at the one–one individual nurse–patient level. Thus, whilst nurses frequently bemoaned the fact that the dietary advice offered to individual patients was often contradicted by the food delivered to these patients at mealtimes, they were not involved in planning for health promotion policy on such issues. In addition, there was a lack of collaborative work with others on health issues in the spirit of a health promotion approach. Individual wards seemed to be isolated units – nurses were often unaware of developments on other wards and complained of a lack of involvement with those working in the community, so that work begun with patients in the hospital could be followed up after their discharge.

A further finding was that although there was some evidence of a participatory approach to care on two case study wards, more generally a participatory or collaborative approach to care with patients was lacking. This was evident in numerous examples of tape recorded nurse–patient interactions. Information and advice giving were frequently characterised by a 'top-down' approach rather than by an exploration of the patient's agenda and equity and collaboration.

> Try not to overeat when you get home as that's normally the cause of people putting weight on, and you do find that a lot of ladies do because they go home and they're not as active as they usually are, yet they're eating the same high calorie foods you would need if you're doing full-time work . . . It's just through eating the wrong foods . . . plus you get really bored when you're sitting at home as well and you just tend to nibble. Try and rally your family round to help you with all your cleaning and washing and everything at first . . . Do try and have a rest in an afternoon, it does help you a lot you know, even if you seem to be resting all the time.

In other instances, it seemed that patients' cues to participate were not always being responded to by nurses. The following example illustrates this and is taken from a nursing bedside handover:

NURSE   I think we're just going on to test your urine. X explained about testing urine didn't she?
PATIENT   I normally do that at home.

NURSE   You do that at home.
PATIENT Yes.
NURSE   Fine.
PATIENT I do that at home.
NURSE   Right, OK. So we'll be doing that twice a day now.

The data indicated that often nurses were operating with an underlying medical model of care and were maintaining the traditional unequal balance of power between 'nurse' and 'patient' roles. Patients were not treated as equal participants in care, but as subordinates, which is contrary to a health promotion approach. In addition, other central concepts and activities were absent from nurses' practice. Nurses did not appear to be involved in empowering patients, fostering self-esteem or encouraging decision-making skills. Again, this is a finding in practice which is closely linked to their perceptions, as outlined above.

Conclusion

To summarise, the study's findings indicate that nurses' perceptions of the concepts of health education and health promotion are closely linked to the way in which they are developing their practice at ward level. That is, both perceptions and practice are characterised by an illness-oriented, one–one approach with a lack of recognition or enactment of many of the central tenets of current health education and health promotion philosophy. The findings suggest that nurses are currently operating with ideologies which closely equate with the traditional or medical model-derived types outlined in the literature. Downie, Fyfe and Tannahill (1990) propose that the traditional approach is characterised by activity aimed at disease prevention rather than positive health and emphasises *physical* health as opposed to social and mental facets. Social and political determinants of health are neglected and activity is targeted at individuals, whilst the collective dimension of health is not addressed. Similar ideas underlie what Tones, Tilford and Robinson (1990) call the 'preventive' model of health education. They suggest that this is derived from the medical model and its goal is to persuade the *individual* to take responsible decisions whilst ignoring the real socio-political roots of ill health. These approaches have an individualistic, physical, illness-oriented focus and are similar to the perceptions and practice of the nurses described above. Possible explanations for these findings were identified, such as hospital nurses' lack of educational exposure to necessary health education and promotion concepts and skills, and their struggle to move away from the medical model of care.

This chapter has highlighted nurses' interpretations of the concepts of health education and health promotion, their role in this and its relationship to practice. Whilst the direction of influence between perceptions and practice may be two-way (i.e. nurses' practice and conditions of work may equally colour their perceptions), it seems clear that if practice is to move forward towards the comprehensive vision that health promotion represents, then nurses' interpretations of what it is that they think they should be doing in its name will need to be addressed.

References

Collins, L. (1984). Concepts of health education: a study of four professional groups. *Journal of the Institute of Health Education, 22,* 3, 81–8.

Department of Health (1989). *A Strategy for Nursing.* A report of the Steering Committee. Department of Health Nursing Division: London.

Downie, R. S. Fyfe, C. and Tannahill, A. (1990). *Health Promotion: Models and Values.* Oxford Medical Publications: Oxford.

Gott, M. and O'Brien, M. (1990). *The Role of the Nurse in Health Promotion: Policies, Perspectives, and Practice.* Report of a 2 year project funded by the Department of Health, London.

Latter, S., Macleod Clark, J., Wilson-Barnett, J. and Maben, J. (1992). Health education in nursing: perceptions of practice in acute settings. *Journal of Advanced Nursing, 17,* 1, 164–72.

Nutbeam, D. (1984). Health education in the National Health Service: the differing perspectives of community physicians and health education officers. *Health Education Journal, 43,* 4, 115–19.

Rawson, D. and Grigg, C. (1988). *Purpose and Practice in Health Education.* South Bank Polytechnic/HEA: London.

RCN (1989). *Into the Nineties: Promoting Professional Excellence.* Royal College of Nursing: London.

Saunders, R. P. (1988). What is health promotion? *Health Education, 19* (5), 14–18.

Tones, K., Tilford, S. and Robinson, Y. (1990). *Health Education: Effectiveness and Efficiency.* Chapman & Hall: London.

10 Opportunities for health education: an analysis of nurse–client interactions in acute areas

Karen Jones

Introduction

Communication between nurse and patient can have a profound impact on the achievement of effective health education practice. This relationship is explored using raw project data (Macleod Clark *et al.*, 1992) of nurse–patient interactions.

The term health education was operationalised for this project (see Chapters 8 & 9) by breaking it down into five categories: information giving, patient participation, family and friends' participation in care, patient education, and healthy lifestyle advice. Tones *et al.* (1990) suggest that health education is a prerequisite in all health promotion programmes: 'It's [health education] function is to influence health choices, its more radical role is to influence the adoption of healthy public policies by raising awareness of the issues in question' (ibid., p. 4).

Background

Education for health is an essential part of today's society, with increasing emphasis being placed on the health education potential of the nurse's role. Clients expect to be more involved in decisions about their health care and want to learn about maintaining and improving their own health, while the number of elderly, chronically sick and seriously ill with degenerative disorders, continue to increase the demands for appropriate intervention. This becomes increasingly relevant when we are told that only 20 per cent of Western ailments are now able to be cured (O'Neil, 1983).

Growing emphasis on health promotion in nursing brings new

demands on nurses' ability to communicate. With Project 2000 the nurse is now expected to care for patients using a perspective which enhances health instead of responding purely to sickness. Demands on nurses' ability to communicate will intensify as we move away from the medical model approach to nursing.

Good communication is fundamental to successful health education. Ewles and Simnett (1992) believe there is a need for clear unambiguous two-way constructive exchanges without distortion of message between when it is given and when it is received. The fundamental aim of health education, they state, is best achieved by working in 'non-judgemental partnership, seeking to build on people's existing knowledge and experience and move them towards autonomy and empower them to take responsibility and feel positive'.

Communication is central to effective health education; for health education to be effective it must meet the needs defined by the patient, and for the nurse to elicit these needs she must be skilled in communicating. If nurses are to move forward research is now needed to examine 'real' encounters to gain a precise assessment of current practice, in order to identify the needs of the nurse, to enable her to begin to meet those of the patient.

Discussion from the case study findings

The actual findings from practice fitted into four of the five categories of activity representing health education practice, as operationalised. Throughout these categories examples are taken from admission, bedside handover and discharge procedures. There is no discussion concerning family or friend participation in care, this is due to its apparent scarcity within the acute clinical environments explored in this project.

It was seen from the interactions between nurses and patients that skilled communication remains for the majority a theoretical concept, as does prevention and promotion of positive health. Even where health education and health promotion were beginning to be integrated into practice, these were found to be largely 'illness-oriented' activities. Let us now look at the findings which underpin such conclusions.

The first category was that of 'information giving'. This was found to be the dominant form of nurse health education practice. However, the range in quality and type given, in addition to the evidence of missed opportunities, may go some way to explain patients' continued dissatisfaction with the information received whilst in hospital. Information given tended to revolve around the ward itself (orientation information), procedures (preprocedural information) and surgery (preoperative information).

Not all nurses offered this type of health education to patients spontaneously, many responded to patients' questions whilst others did not venture information when asked or given a 'cue' by the patient. For example, during an admission, the nurse was asking the patient about her family:

NURSE   Right, right. And do they know what is wrong with you?
PATIENT Well, they know I've come in for this investigation thing, like you know, and this wire, it is something to do with a wire isn't it, going up into the heart?
NURSE   Right. So apart from your husband, is there any other person we can contact? (Taped admission)

Here the patient's needs were not addressed despite her direct question to the nurse. The nurse instead seems intent on obtaining information dictated by the admission form. This leads us on to the finding that the admission procedure itself was seen by nurses in general to be a good opportunity for health education. However, the way admissions were conducted frequently reflected an approach where the sole aim appeared to be collecting information and filling in the forms. Communication was often confined to details of physical care only, with little attention to the patient's psychological or social needs; a finding that is characteristic of the 'medical model' approach to care.

A lack of communication skills training is often cited as one reason for nurses failing to recognise patient cues or address their needs. Not only were direct 'cues' often missed by the quality of the interactions varied greatly. If open questions were asked, they were frequently immediately closed again.

This next example did seem to reflect a 'more' skilful and knowledgeable approach to communication. Here the nurse is offering a patient information, in preparation for an impending procedure:

NURSE   They keep taking different pictures as they go along, so they know they're going into the right place. OK?
PATIENT Lovely, yes, I can sleep tonight now . . . might get some sleep.
NURSE   Has that eased your mind a little bit?
PATIENT Yes, it has, a little bit, thanks. You see, you say what I don't know I don't grieve, but what you imagine can make it worse, can't it?
NURSE   Yes. Your mind can play havoc with you.

To conclude then, analysis revealed that information was often sought by patients rather than spontaneously offered by nurses.

Let us now move to the second category for discussion, that of patient participation. Patients often expressed a desire to participate in their care despite, rather than because of, nurses' communications. Some attempted to participate almost against the odds. Examples showed other characteristic features of the bedside handover, where nurses often appeared to talk to each other over the patient, while the patient often had more accurate information than the nurse who was handing over.

One particular observation records the patient's surprise when invited to participate. An example from the observation notes illustrates this:

> NURSE   All I've written there is a little plan about what we're going to do, that you've come in with chest pain and that you're going to have grafts done. There you are read that and see what you think.

The nurse puts the folder on the patient's bed, and the patient replies:

> PATIENT   Am I allowed to read it?
> NURSE   Yes, of course you are, it's for you to read.
> PATIENT   Years ago you would have got your hands chopped off if you'd have touched that.

On this particular ward the researchers found that patients were encouraged to participate in their care and to have some control over their stay on the ward. Documentation was kept in folders at the end of the patient's bed and nurse folders had notices attached: 'Please do not read these notes without permission from the patient.' Some nurses were seen by the researchers to ask patients before looking in these folders.

From the same ward, here is an example of how a bedside handover did become an opportunity for patients to participate in their care. This example identifies a more skilled approach:

> NURSE 1   Right, X's looking after you this afternoon.
> PATIENT   Yes, all right.
> NURSE 1   OK, um. I'm going off shortly. Do you just want to tell her how you've been.
> PATIENT   Well, I've been quite well. I had a bath yesterday, had a wash today, and general . . . getting better. I go to the toilet all right and very well.
> NURSE 2   Yeah.
> NURSE 1   Do you think that you are generally improving X?
> PATIENT   I definitely am, very much so, I'm going home tomorrow.
> NURSE 2   Great.

Other examples can be found in which patient participation in care was minimal, indeed there was evidence to suggest that care plans and evaluations were written with minimal consultation with the patients.

The researchers found bedside handovers were often characterised by the 'role playing' of 'nurse' and 'patient', such that the patient adopted a passive, submissive, almost childlike, role whilst the nurse was the dominant or 'parental' figure. Such an approach resulted in a hierarchical interaction between the 'expert' and 'non-expert'. This is the antithesis of a health promoting approach in which collaboration, equal participation and empowerment are paramount.

Thirdly, we will discuss the area of patient education. The extent to which nurses had integrated patient education into practice again showed great variance. A more formal and planned session was observed and tape recorded in which the nurse was educating the patient about her medications prior to discharge. Here the nurse displays skills in both communication and teaching. She uses a drug card as a teaching tool, picks up the patient's cues, and is prepared to leave her agenda and follow that of the patient, whilst assessing the patient's knowledge.

NURSE   So when would you take this, do you think?
PATIENT   Well, if I ever get that pain there. But some days I only get it once a day or not at all. I don't take it if I've got no pain.
NURSE   That's right. And do you have a rest at the same time?
PATIENT   Yes, I always sit down for about ten minutes, quarter of an hour after I usually get that pain if I've done a bit of hoovering, you know.
NURSE   That's right. And you were saying yesterday that you know how much you can do and when you've got to stop.

The above example did not appear indicative of the general level of patient education found in the acute areas. The majority of examples consisted of planned sessions which were predominantly 'nurse led'. There seemed, in general, little integration of patient education on a spontaneous level.

Lastly, we will consider the sharing of healthy lifestyle advice. There was some evidence of this, but overall it would not appear to be considered comprehensive or substantive from the evidence of the transcripts. The majority of these illustrate how nurse–patient communication was often 'nurse led' and dominated by the physical concerns underpinning the medical model approach to nursing care. We would do well to remember the earlier quotation from Ewles and Simnett (1992) where they state that the fundamental aim of health education is best achieved by working in 'non-judgemental partnership'. If nurses persist in following the 'medical model' approach this aim becomes a remote possibility. It is perhaps to Project 2000 that we now look to redress the balance.

Conclusions

In sharing the above interactions I do not want to give the impression of seeing the nurse as the prime cause of poor communication and health promoting activity. In reading through the transcripts I saw many reminders of my own practice and the missed opportunities for health education in the clinical area. Health education has moved on and now nurses must do the same, but they need to be helped to do so. Nurses need to understand the 'philosophy' upon which they are now being expected to base their practice.

To 'empower' others it is essential initially to feel empowered yourself; to understand another's perspective you must have a clear idea about your own. This is supported by the finding that areas where health education appeared to be integrated into practice were environments where the management was democratic, where nurses felt empowered and autonomous within their own practice, where organisation of care provided continuity, and where the philosophy of the ward and its staff was one of equality and collaboration.

If we are serious about promoting health it is essential that all nurses are helped to develop communication skills needed to act as facilitators. As horizons of nursing practice changes so the challenges to our communication skills will increase.

References

Ewles, L. and Simnett, I. (1992). *Promoting Health – A Practical Guide*. Scutari Press: London.

Macleod Clark, J., Wilson-Barnett, J., Latter, S. and Maben, J. (1992). Health education and health promotion in nursing: a study of practice in acute areas. Unpublished research report, Department of Health.

O'Neill, P. (1983). *Health Crisis 2000*. WHO: Geneva.

Tones, K., Tilford, S., and Robinson, Y. (1990). *Health Education – Effectiveness and Efficiency*. Chapman & Hall: London.

11 Lay participation in care: threat to the status quo

Julienne Meyer

Introduction

This chapter draws from case study data obtained from research exploring the introduction of lay participation in care within the context of a hospital ward environment. Using illuminative evaluation strategies (Parlett and Hamilton, 1977) and an action research approach (Elliott, 1991), I worked together with a multidisciplinary team, on a general medical ward in a London teaching hospital, for a period of one year in an attempt to foster practice which would involve patients and their family/friends in care, with a view to better preparation for discharge. A multimethod approach to data collection was taken including in-depth interviews, questionnaires and participant observation recorded in daily field notes. I held weekly team meetings with participants to feedback findings and plan and evaluate action strategies. Whilst at the end of this period positive changes could be claimed, the process of innovation was extremely slow and various factors which hindered and facilitated developments will be discussed in this chapter. The slowness of organisational change in the health service has been described in other case studies by Stocking (1985) but this study specifically relates to initiatives to develop health promotion roles and describes the inertia in detail as health professionals were forced to challenge the status quo of traditional practice.

Definition

Lay participation in care is concerned with the involvement of non-professionals in care. McEwen *et al.* (1983) describe participation in care as

> the process whereby a person can function on his or her own behalf in the maintenance and promotion of health, the prevention of disease, the detection, treatment and care of illness and adaptation

to continuing disability. It may occur independently of, or within, the existing system of care and extends to activities performed on behalf of others (e.g. family participation) and in the planning, management and evaluation of health care provision. (McEwen *et al.*, 1983)

McEwen *et al.* identify the main underlying concepts involved in participation as 'self-help', 'demedicalisation or deprofessionalisation' and 'democratisation'. These concepts generally underpin modern day understandings of health promotion and it is not surprising that lay participation in care is described as an important thread of health promotion (Kickbush, 1981). True participation in care is thus concerned with patient empowerment. It acknowledges a change in relationship between the professional and lay person emphasising partnership in care.

Within nursing, partnership is currently a key issue as specified in the Strategy for Nursing document (Department of Health, 1989) and underpins the new courses in nurse education (United Kingdom Central Council for Nursing, 1986). Within the health service the concept is further promulgated in the form of 'patient as consumer' (Department of Health, 1992; Secretaries of State for Health, 1989).

However, concern has been shown over the interest of health professionals in participation in care and suggestions made that in some cases participation is viewed as mere tokenism (Brownlea, 1987) or manipulation towards compliance with medical treatments and not true partnership in care (Brearley, 1990). Furthermore, it has been suggested by some nurse researchers that patients may not wish to participate in care and find themselves coerced as reluctant collaborators (Waterworth and Luker, 1990). A review of the literature reveals much rhetoric with few empirical studies (Brooking, 1986).

Whilst there is insufficient research evidence to support current developments, it is recognised that due to changing health care contexts, maintaining the status quo is not an option (Dingwall *et al.*, 1988). Lay participation in care is seen as part of the new nursing professional ideology (Beardshaw and Robinson, 1990) and practitioners are being urged to develop approaches to health care based on partnership. In view of these recommended changes in practice, I felt that a case study was needed to explore in detail the issues and problems resulting from such initiatives. I decided to use an action research approach in the case study for several reasons. First, action research focuses on the process and outcome of change. Given that lay participation in care is an approach to care which is hard to define in practical terms, I felt that a study which looked at the development of these ideas in practice might be more useful than an evaluation of an institution claiming to have initiated such a scheme. Second, action research is practice oriented and as such deals with reality. I thought this to be particularly important given that previous research had identified that whilst health professionals felt positive towards the concept of lay participation in care, the use of theoretical scales to measure complex phenomena had been questioned (Brooking, 1986). By using an action research approach I believed I would be in a better position to explore with health professionals their real attitudes towards lay participation in care when confronting the concept in their everyday practice. Third, action research is perceived as being part of a new paradigm of research which emphasises doing research *with* and *for* people rather than *on* people (Reason and Rowan, 1981). I therefore felt it held the same philosophical underpinnings as lay participation in care and was consequently the most appropriate way to examine the concept. Furthermore, given that more traditional types of nursing research had been criticised for their general lack of relevance to practice (Greenwood, 1984), I hoped that by giving participants more control over the research process itself findings would be more accessible and useful to them.

This chapter does not address the issues related to the process of doing an action research study, but presents the findings related to the health professionals' understanding and experience of trying to promote lay participation in care within the context of a hospital setting. The findings will be presented using Stocking's framework, namely the influence of the environment, the characteristics of the innovation and the people in the process (Stocking, 1985).

The influence of the environment

Given that societal views can affect the acceptability of innovations, I shall begin by reviewing those findings which indicated that the health professionals in the study did not feel committed to the concept of lay participation in care, despite articulating positive views in theory. It is argued that some of their reservations were due to their own lack of conceptual understanding and a belief that lay participation in care was not a socially accepted phenomenon.

The influence of societal views on professional perceptions

Data gathered at interview from the multidisciplinary team revealed that the health professionals had a limited understanding of lay participation in care. Health professionals seemed to find it difficult to articulate what was meant by lay participation in care and there was little mention of the concepts related to health promotion such as self-help, patient empowerment, equality and partnership. There also appeared to be a lack of understanding of the philosophical underpinnings such as demedicalisation, deprofessionalisation and democratisation.

It was interesting that whilst health professionals expressed overall favourable attitudes to participation in care, through the Patient and Family Participation in Care Scale (Brooking, 1986), they none the less indicated more negative views at interview and were clearly not committed to the concept in the reality of practice. Health professionals did not appear to engage with patients as equals and the traditional medical model of practice was very much in evidence. Attempts to move towards more client centred approaches proved problematic. Whilst the professionals did not appear to want to relinquish their authority and control, the patients themselves lacked an expectation to be treated any differently. In fact this lack of expectation to be involved in care inhibited professionals from being more committed to the concept. For instance, concern was expressed by health professionals that lay people might not want to participate in care and that they would feel guilty offloading their work on others. Involvement in care was seen very much in terms of the sharing of practical nursing tasks and viewed as a potentially unwelcome burden on lay people. As one of the nurses commented:

> I've got my doubts whether the average person in the street will want to come into hospital and start looking after their relatives and carry on at home. I think that as well as the doubts, they may well feel that we're trying to transfer our responsibilities onto them to save money – maybe it's a political thing. They might say why should we do this when you're paid to do it, we've paid our stamps . . . because people tend to use the social state, don't they, to full advantage now.

Van den Heuval (1980) would argue that behind this notion of lay participation in care is the historical legacy of bureaucratic cost effectiveness and economic stringency as opposed to the more feminist historical legacy of equality and human rights. Clearly societal views influenced the professionals desire to facilitate lay people to participate in care. They felt suspicious of the motives behind the study and did not appear to comprehend the more humanistic perspective of involvement.

The lack of commitment towards the professionals changing their practice should also be understood in the light of the wider environmental context of that time. The next section will look at what was going on in the hospital at the time and then the local environment of the ward will be explored.

The hospital context

During the period of the study the hospital was under pressure to improve efficiency and service to patients while keeping within a reducing budget. It was in the middle of the post-Griffiths turmoil when major changes were occurring in the National Health Service and in particular senior nurses were feeling very much under threat (Robinson *et al.*, 1989). It was at the time of the regrading exercise and nurses at all levels were being asked to look at their job descriptions, roles and responsibilities (perhaps for the first time) and were feeling undervalued with many going to appeal. On top of this, Project 2000 was on the agenda and participants were feeling apprehensive as to where they were going to fit into this major educational reform. Within the hospital the workload had generally increased with the fixed establishment not accommodating the increase in demand for care. A local hospital, down the road, had been closed and posts were being ring fenced for the future amalgamation of staff from the two separate sites which represented a mixing of two different cultures. The ward clerks were in the middle of a two-year dispute and working to rule, the cleaning had gone out to tender and was proving inadequate and the staff were having to contend with support services trying in vain to run at a five-day week. Generally, morale was extremely low with people adjusting to new ideas, concepts and roles and working under less than adequate conditions. Pressure was exerted to reduce waiting lists and there was a movement towards thinking about trust status. A top down approach to change was being forced and it left health professionals feeling under enormous stress.

Given the environment, it is little wonder that the health professionals felt suspicious of the rationale for participation in care. It is also not surprising that they did not have the energies for innovating change.

Whilst one might question the choice of ward/hospital for innovating change, I believe the environment was no different from many other hospital environments at that point in history. Considering that so much change was being forced from above, it could be argued that a bottom up approach to change might have empowered participants to cope better with their situation. By taking a non-directive facilitatory role, I hoped not to force my ideas on the participants but to enable them to examine their practice and reflect upon new ways of giving care, more in line with future health care needs.

The ward

The ward was clearly run on a functional rather than developmental model. Routinised care was administered in a task-oriented manner.

On the medical side, the housemen who were allocated to the ward for a three-month rotation hid behind routine tasks to keep their heads above water. They found it hard to engage with the project ideas, being pushed in at the deep end at the beginning of their allocation with little handover or management support and development from their superiors. By the time they came to the end of their allocation they were just about coping with the routine nature of their work and had started to see for themselves the importance of lay participation in care. The transient nature of their work inhibited them from fostering more patient-centred approaches to care. Their motivating force was to get on to the next rung of their career ladder. As one houseman said:

> Oh, I don't think you want to upset the kind of people like consultants, I mean I wouldn't dream of saying, 'I don't think you should take students on ward rounds because it upsets patients . . .' they'd say, 'Don't tell me, I'm a consultant' . . . I wouldn't get a good reference . . . I think you do have to observe . . . routines and . . . my job . . . At times there is almost too much to do and I just get on with sticking needles in people and making sure they've signed their consents when they go to theatre, but I don't see it as kind of holistic . . . maybe I should, but I just don't think I have the time or resources available to think more about the patient and his environment.

Nurses similarly were set in old routine and task-oriented habits and found it difficult to change. The ward was not seen as a good ward-learning environment for learners and students complained that they were not adequately monitored or supported by staff. Staff at all levels indicated that they felt generally unsupported by their colleagues and the ward was seen as being disorganised and suffering from poor communication. Within the team health professionals were not sharing information, not using each other's skills or appreciating the different roles and contributions of other team members.

Data from the initial interviews with the multidisciplinary team suggested that before lay participation in care could be introduced, more fundamental issues needed to be addressed in terms of the way the ward was organised to offer such an individualised approach to care. It was suggested by participants that a modified form of primary nursing was needed to encourage nurses to take responsibility for forming closer relationships with patients and their family/friends in order to offer lay participation in care. Furthermore, it was suggested that before participation could be offered to lay people there needed to be more participation within the multidisciplinary team itself.

Not only did new systems of work need to be set up in order to foster a more individualised approach to care, but health professionals also discovered that lay participation in care was not part of their normal practice. First, professionals did not appear to see patients in a holistic way and were often unaware of their patients' social circumstances. As one houseman said:

> I'll never forget, someone died, and it just didn't dawn on me to ring the relatives, you just don't think about those sort of things. I mean I do now, but when you first start, because as a student you have nothing to do with the social situation with the patient, it's all like . . . well they've got this or that, what does it mean . . . you're thinking more about the clinical side of the patient rather than every other implication.

Even when relatives visited the ward, there was a lack of contact between them and the professionals. This lack of contact sometimes led to inappropriate discharges being arranged. Visitors appeared to have no role on the ward and were often perceived as a problem by getting in the way or by being too demanding. Where families did get involved with care, it was generally at their initiation rather than being professionally led. Once participation in care had been initiated, professionals often formed close and meaningful relationships with the patients and their family/friends and it was interesting to note that those who did initiate this type of contact tended to be the family/friends of AIDS patients or those with terminally ill relatives.

Family/friends generally did not appear to expect to be involved in hospital care. Often they would withdraw from the bedside when a ward round approached. They appeared frightened to ask questions or to be seen as interfering. This behaviour was often reinforced by the professionals' response to them. As one nurse said:

> I mean, you see it all the time. I think if you go on a ward round the relatives will always leave the bedside and the doctors never encourage them to stay unless there's something particular that they think is relevant you know, . . . how are you going to manage at home, sort of thing, or a particular question they want to ask. But . . . they're quite happy for the relative to leave, you know, and on occasions when the relative has perhaps been a little more aggressive and not left, I've always perceived that some of the medical staff and the nursing staff have felt uncomfortable by the relative's presence.

On the ward there was a lack of patient education. Professionals tended to control information and keep patients in the dark. Patients did not have access to notes, care plans were not jointly discussed and the day to day information such as results of blood tests, changes in treatment regimes, etc. were not routinely shared with patients. Nurses tended to leave information giving to the doctors or get patients referred to specialists (e.g. diabetic nurse). Health education was rarely carried out and when health advice was given to patients it tended to be prescriptive and given in an authoritarian manner.

From the above it can be seen that the introduction of lay participation in care constituted a major change in practice for this multidisciplinary team and it is little wonder that the process of change was slow. The next section will examine the characteristics of the innovation.

Characteristics of the innovation

Rogers (1983) identifies five particular attributes that affect the uptake of an innovation: relative advantage, compatibility, complexity, trialability and observability. These attributes will be examined in turn in relation to the project.

Relative advantage

This concerns the degree to which the innovation is perceived as better than the one that precedes it.

As mentioned before health professionals were not totally committed to the concept of lay participation in care. They found it hard to think of ways in which lay people could be encouraged to participate more and were reluctant to relinquish their professional roles. As one staff nurse revealed:

> I think it's really a good idea. I think the one thing you have to bear in mind is perhaps for the relatives not to take on too much . . . and at the same time I think it's difficult, or I find it difficult myself, to know what sort of tasks to give them to do and what not to give them to, and sometimes I find myself hanging on to it all because that's my role and you know it's easy to hide behind the nurse's role. I can do all this and get on and do it, and it is more difficult and perhaps takes longer to involve them in care.

Health professionals questioned whether in general patients were going to be suitable for this approach to health care. Patients were thought to have no relatives, be confused, depressed or too dependent and sick to participate in care. Professionals expressed reluctance to pass over their responsibility to lay people, fearing the legal implications of lay people doing harm on the basis of little knowledge. Other concerns focused on the changes as being a threat to professional practice. Medical staff were reluctant to allow the development of non-medical ideas on the ward. Aromatherapy was viewed with scepticism as being unscientific and health promotion leaflets needed to be vetted for fear of conflicting messages.

Professionals also showed a lack of commitment to lay participation in care on account of it requiring too much effort on their part to implement, being time consuming and potentially more stressful for professionals having to deal more closely with the public. This made some professionals feel particularly vulnerable:

> I think all of us are probably a little reluctant to allow relatives, non-members of our professions, to be involved in patient care . . . We might tend to think, right, things are probably going to get messed up, our routine is going to be messed up, we'll have to share all our idiosyncrasies and our frustrations and all the rest with the relatives and they'll see what we are really like, whereas we want to retain our respectability and so there may be quite a few hidden reasons why the flesh is weak.

Compatibility

Compatibility concerns the degree to which the innovation is perceived as consistent with the existing values, past experiences and needs of potential adopters. As already discussed, health professionals had some concerns about the ethics of involving lay people in hospital care and found that it challenged their previous modes of work. For many they found it threatening to have their status quo challenged and did not welcome the move towards a new professional model of care. The nurse in charge saw these developments as taking her away from bedside nursing and into an area of management she did not feel equipped to deal with. She did not want to relinquish her authoritarian role as nurse in charge and move towards an educative/supportive role as ward coordinator. By refusing to do this she actively inhibited the professional development of her staff in augmenting their educative/supportive roles with patients. Some staff were similarly dissatisfied with the direction in which nursing was going. Several nurses identified that they had been just coming to work to do a job and felt no commitment to the development of professional nursing. As one nurse said:

> I've never felt like a dedicated nurse . . . There's the type who are innovative and always thinking of new ideas and they're dynamic, then I suppose there's a type like me who just likes to do their work, do what's needed and leave it at that. They're not exactly keen . . . The non-dynamic ones, I think, must want to do their job, enjoy

themselves while they're there and go home . . . well, me, I haven't read up an awful lot at home. I haven't done any work outside.

Other staff nurses were more enthusiastic about the developments in nursing and wanted to be involved and have the opportunity of improving their practice. As one nurse said:

> I'm very strongly in favour of primary nursing . . . I've been here for two years now and I've never been appraised. No one has ever said, you are doing this right, you could improve here, you could improve there, so I don't know where I'm going wrong. I have no confidence in what I'm doing and people say the same thing. I mean there are a lot of newly qualified staff nurses on and they don't know what they're doing right and what they're doing wrong.

This difference in opinion over the compatibility of the innovation with people's desire for practice led to a non-cohesive team pulling in different directions and getting nowhere fast.

Complexity

Complexity concerns the degree to which the innovation is perceived as relatively difficult to understand and to use.

It has already been mentioned that health professionals found it hard to articulate what was meant by lay participation in care. The doctors in the study saw it more as a nursing issue rather than anything that should particularly concern them. In terms of it being difficult to use, generally health professionals found they lacked the skills and confidence to develop educative/supportive roles with lay people. As one house officer commented:

> Talking to patients about diet . . . I've realised, my God, I don't know what I'm talking about, and I keep saying, well, I'll get you some leaflets but I can never find them, never ever . . . We know the medical side of things but you don't know what common knowledge is.

Another nurse said:

> With the health education leaflet, for the first time, I was sitting down talking to a patient, talking about their illness, what to look for, and I didn't realise how little they knew and how bad an educator I was. I've never had to do it before. I've actually sat down and educated someone and I realised I was quite bad at it. I couldn't put things across.

Talking to lay people was often seen as a low priority task and delegated to junior staff who often did not have the experience or expertise to cope well when dealing with difficult situations, such as sharing poor prognoses or explaining things in lay terms. The lack of role models meant that participants had to learn the hard way and were probably put off engaging with lay people as a result. A doctor reflected on the inadequacies in medical training in this respect:

> I think the reflection on the training comes when you see what happens to you as a houseman . . . a lot of them are completely shell shocked, totally and utterly shell shocked because suddenly they have to be involved in a personal way, not just from exhaustion, which is part of it, but also death. They're not trained to cope with death and then you tell them they've got to cope with death, either you've seen it as a student and been part of it or you haven't, it just sort of happens, and telling relatives. Students are never with me when I'm telling relatives what's going to happen, maybe occasionally but very rare.

Nurses similarly found it difficult to teach and support learners and as a result tended to cling to tasks rather than develop more educative/ supportive roles. They found it hard to break old habits and practices and develop new skills. Nurses who coped better with the change tended to be more assertive and better able to deal with working in a democratic way both with lay people and their colleagues. For others the concept was too complex really to comprehend and utilise.

Trialability

Trialability concerned the degree to which the innovation could be experimented with on a limited basis. Trialability in this study was severely limited by the transient nature of the workforce. Being a teaching hospital, staff were often rotating around the wards to gain experience and staying for only short periods of time. During the course of the study eighty new staff (including nurse learners) joined the team and eighty-five left, and there were only five members of staff remaining in post at the end of the study who were there at the beginning. This transiency made continuity of care difficult and innovatory work almost impossible. The transient nature of the workforce made it difficult to establish a cohesive multidisciplinary team that could work together to make change. As one paramedic said:

> I was probably there too for short a time to grasp hold of the whole thing really, because I was probably more interested in getting to know about the physio side rather than any other side. So to be

quite honest I probably didn't take much notice of what the other multidisciplinary team . . . how they . . . what they were actually doing as part of your research thing, so I didn't probably really notice what was going on.

Observability

Observability concerns the degree to which the results of an innovation are observable to others. Progress was slow and whilst it could be claimed that positive change was achieved, the results were not very visible and led staff to feeling disillusioned with the lack of progress. As one nurse said:

I was quite enthusiastic to begin with and, I don't know, but it just seemed as if everyone was hitting their heads against a brick wall from the beginning to the end and just more and more difficulties were coming up – and I began to lose faith . . . Until I moved to another ward I didn't realise how much I had actually learnt from x. Whereas moving to another ward and now being able to come out at meetings and things with something we had discussed on x, and saying, 'Did you know that we can get leaflets on this and that?' . . . then you suddenly realise that we actually did go quite a long way towards helping our patients more.

Staff lacked a confidence about their own professional practice and before any of them could get out of their rut, they required considerable time and effort in personal and professional development which was only made possible by a change in the nurse in charge during the study. This second nurse in charge proved to be a more dynamic and enthusiastic leader and by caring for and supporting her colleagues was able to lead her staff out of a situation of staff conflict and inertia.

The final part of this chapter will go on to discuss the people in the process.

People in the process

This section will look at the power relations within the multidisciplinary team and discuss how this affected the innovation. It will also look at the importance of the role of the ward sister as a dynamic leader in managing change.

Medical dominance became a key issue in this study, which set out to use democratic processes in decision-making. However, in multidisciplinary team meetings medical staff (in particular senior members) dominated discussions. Junior medical staff, nurses and paramedical staff appeared reluctant to engage in debate for fear of upsetting their perceived superiors. Even when they did not agree with decisions made they would rather express this informally to me rather than in formal meetings. For instance, one paramedic said, with reference to the consultant:

> I think people are just slightly intimidated; they don't want to say what they really feel in front of somebody who might be in a position to criticise them, or to say, well, why do you say that. I don't think that. You don't want to get into a confrontation situation with your superiors, I suppose.

Whilst the consultant clearly saw himself as head of patient care, he did not see himself as a manager of change in ward practice. This was seen as the role and responsibility of the nurse in charge who was expected to monitor the junior medical staff as well as the nursing staff.

> I think it has to come from the ward sister who is there all the time. I think if you have a ward sister who believes this is a thing to do and can motivate her nurses, this will be very important in motivating the housemen because probably if you look at it, the sister and the nurses have as much, if not more contact with them than the consultants, and certainly the senior registrar. So I think that could be a valuable way of educating the housemen as well as integrating them into the system.

However, the hierarchical power structures meant that if the senior medical staff did not actively support and monitor the implementation of project ideas, junior medical staff would neglect their responsibilities in the change process. The expectation that the sister would manage junior medical staff as well as her own nurses was a hidden phenomenon, as she did not necessarily perceive she had a responsibility to do so. As a result, housemen were expected to work in an autonomous way and were not given much support or orientation into the ways of ward practice. This lack of involvement by senior medical staff with changing practice on the ward meant that it was in many ways in their own best interests to maintain the status quo. Whilst verbally supporting the project they exhibited all the signs of Schon's dynamic conservatism (Schon, 1971).

As with the junior medical staff, the nurses and paramedical staff were reluctant to change practice without the full support of the senior medical staff. Within the nursing team the same power relations existed in relation to the nurse in charge of the ward. Her support and leadership was essential for junior nurses to feel able to change their practice. This clearly demonstrates the importance of the role of the ward sister in leading multidisciplinary change. Within weeks of the second ward sister being on the ward, the multidisciplinary team were working more cohesively and some of the project ideas were being implemented more successfully. The second sister was perceived as a quietly dynamic and enthusiastic leader committed to professional nursing. She was well educated (was just finishing a part-time degree), research minded and capable of being reflective and self-critical. She was not threatened by change and was confident and assertive in the multidisciplinary team. She encouraged open and honest relationships and created a supportive and caring environment for her staff. She saw her role as being facilitator of the other staff's professional development and acted as a role model and adviser in dealing with patients and their family and friends.

Whilst this second ward sister affected change on the ward that was evaluated positively by participants, she would not claim to have been able to bring the team to a point of being able to offer lay participation in care. She struggled to make the changes on the ward at her own personal cost, often working in her own time, largely unsupported by management. She had the strength and confidence to confront issues that had been swept under the carpet in the past, but found the pressures of working in an environment of constant cutbacks frustrating and demotivating. Lack of time, resources and the general inefficiencies of support systems were all key issues she had to deal with. Lay participation in care remained a threat to the status quo, but given all the odds against achieving change one wonders if maintaining the status quo might have been a healthier option for participants.

References

Beardshaw, V. and Robinson, R. (1990). *New for Old? Prospects for Nursing in the 1990s*. King's Fund Institute: London.

Brearley, S. (1990). *Patient Participation: The Literature*. Scutari Press: London.

Brooking, J. (1986). *Patient and Family Participation in Nursing Care: The Development of a Nursing Process Measuring Scale*. Unpublished Ph.D. thesis, University of London.

Brownlea, A. (1987). Participation, myths, realities and prognosis. *Social Science and Medicine*, 25 6, 607–14.

Department of Health (1989). *Strategies for Nursing*. HMSO: London.

Department of Health (1992). *The Health of the Nation*. HMSO: London.

Dingwall, R., Rafferty, A. M. and Webster, C. (1988). *Introduction to the Social History of Nursing*. Routledge: London.

Elliott, J. (1991). *Action Research for Educational Change: Developing Teachers and Teaching*. Open University Press: Milton Keynes.

Greenwood, J. (1984). Nursing research: a position paper. *Journal Of Advanced Nursing*, 9, 77–82.

Kickbush, I. (1981). Involvement in health: a social concept of health education. *International Journal of Health Education, Supplement to volume XXIV* (no. 4).

McEwen, J., Martini, C. J. M. and Wilkins, N. (1983). *Participation in Health.* Croom Helm: London.

Parlett, M. and Hamilton, D. (1977). Evaluation as illumination: a new approach to the study of innovatory programmes, in Hamilton, D., Jenkins, D., King, C., MacDonald, B. and Parlett, M. (eds). *Beyond the Numbers Game.* Macmillan Education: London.

Reason, P. and Rowan, J. (ed.) (1981). *Human Inquiry: A Sourcebook of New Paradigm Research.* John Wiley: Chichester.

Robinson, J., Strong, P. and Elkan, R. (1989). *Griffiths and the Nurses: A National Survey of CNAs* (no. NPS4). Nursing Policy Studies Centre. University of Warwick: Warwick.

Rogers, E. (1983). *Diffusion of Innovations,* 3rd ed. Free Press: New York.

Schon, D. (1971). *Beyond the Stable State.* Random House: London.

Secretaries of State for Health, W., Northern Ireland and Scotland (1989). *Working for Patients.* HMSO (Cmnd 555): London.

Stocking, B. (1985). *Initiative and Inertia: Case Studies in the NHS.* The Nuffield Provincial Hospitals Trust: London.

United Kingdom Central Council for Nursing, M. a. H. V. (1986). *Project 2000: A New Preparation for Practice.* UKCC: London.

Van den Heuval, W. J. A. (1980). The role of the consumer in health policy. *Social Science and Medicine, 14A,* 423–6.

Waterworth, S. and Luker, K. (1990). Reluctant collaborators: do patients want to be involved in decisions concerning care? *Journal of Advanced Nursing, 15,* 971–6.

12 *Hospitalisation and discharge of stroke patients: the relatives' experiences*

Mary Flatley

It is well recognised that stroke can have a devastating effect on the patient, but the effects on the family are less clear cut. Long-term studies of informal carers have identified a fairly high prevalence of depression, emotional reactions, sleep disturbance and social isolation (Greveson *et al.*, 1991). Little research has been carried out on looking at family experiences during rehabilitation. Anderson (1992), in a lengthy study found that in the first few weeks many patients and supporters had high hopes for the effects of rehabilitation, but when interviewed later expressed disappointment at the results. The aim of this study was to explore the experiences of relatives during the time the patient was in hospital and following discharge. A major theme to emerge is that relatives need to understand about the stroke in order to cope with it. One important aspect of this is the relatives role in relation to the progress and recovery of the patient. This chapter focuses on two facets of this role which are related to the concept of health promotion in important ways. These are:

- being informed;
- being involved in care.

Participation in care has been long accepted as an important strand of health promotion. It has many definitions but Brownlea's seems to be the most applicable in this context: 'Participation means getting involved or being allowed to become involved in a decision-making process or the delivery of a service or the evaluation of a service, or even simply to become one of a number of people consulted on an issue or matter' (Brownlea, 1987). Information is assumed to be a prerequisite of participation in care.

Much of the literature focuses on participation in decision-making in doctor–patient relations and the role of information exchange within this. Many of the studies are carried out in an outpatient or community setting. In nursing literature, participation in care has been addressed within the hospital setting mainly in the areas of decision-making and care planning. However, this concept underpins many of the nursing models and processes used in hospital. Rehabilitation is also allied to the idea of patient participation in care with emphasis on the need for patient and relative interaction. However, there is a paucity of research into the practicalities of achieving it within the hospital ward setting.

In Chapter 11 of this book Meyer, using an action research approach, attempted systematically to introduce lay participation in care within an acute medical ward. Professionals felt it was a positive undertaking but there were many barriers to prevent it happening, including medical dominance, conservatism and the sense of being a threat to professional practice. Latter, in Chapter 9, looked at ward sisters' perceptions of health education and health promotion and found that few of them thought participation was a noteable feature. They perceived participation as advantageous mainly with terminally ill or stroke patients.

But what are patients' and relatives' preferences for participation? Waterworth and Luker (1990) found that patients can be reluctant collaborators but they did not address the relatives' perceptions. Much of what is written about these ideas tends to refer to patients and relatives together whereas it is likely that their perceptions and preferences differ.

Methods

This research was based in one district general hospital and one teaching hospital where I identified patients who had been admitted with a first stroke, who had a good prognosis of survival and who had a close relative. I interviewed the relative within two to four weeks of the patient's admission, again within a week to two of the discharge and then about eight to twelve weeks later. Although both places had a designated stroke unit most patients were admitted first to a medical ward and not all were transferred to the stroke units before being discharged. A semi-structured interview was used and the data analysed qualitatively for emerging themes. In all I recruited thirty-six relatives but was not able to carry out second and third interviews on all of them for varying reasons, the main one being the death of the patient.

Being informed

In this study most relatives had very little previous knowledge of strokes. What they knew was related to loss in function in the arm and leg, and facial signs such as a drooping mouth. Many had no knowledge of the possible effects of stroke on speech, swallowing, memory and mood. Previous experience of stroke within the family or with friends led to preconceptions about the outcome. The onset of the stroke was often attributed to a recent event which the patient had found stressful, while a history of high blood pressure or diabetes was also thought to be contributory.

Most people were told of the diagnosis in the accident and emergency department. Many described long periods of waiting which contrasted fiercely with the rush to get to hospital. There was a sense of wanting more information at this time.

Sources of knowledge were varied and numerous:

- Some people had neighbours or friends who were nurses or who had experienced stroke within the family.
- Others went to their GP or were given leaflets about stroke within the hospital, but provision of these was erratic and inconsistent.
- Some obtained leaflets from the Stroke Association.
- One was given a book by a friend.
- One man described how a distant relative who was a doctor had visited the patient in hospital examined him and then reassured the family of his progress.

Types and amounts of knowledge required were varied and individualistic. Almost all relatives expressed a need for further information, mainly concerning causes, what to expect and whether it would happen again.

There seems to be some confusion among relatives about what it is they want to know, and this may affect the kind and number of questions they ask. Individuals appear to fall into an active–passive continuum related to the acquisition of knowledge. Those at the passive end of the spectrum did not seek information. If given verbal or written instructions they were pleased to receive them but would not actively request them from medical or nursing staff. However, they would telephone daily for some sort of progress report but were content, as one man said, 'to leave it in their hands'. Several relatives said that other members of the family asked the questions or the patient kept the relative informed of progress, but some had no expectation of being informed even though they had concerns about how they would cope on discharge. It is possible that for some people this passive approach is a manifestation of the use of denial as a coping mechanism.

Those at the more active end of the scale described themselves as 'always asking questions' or 'wanting to know'. They perceived knowledge of progress and prognosis as a way of preparing themselves for discharge or as a way of coping with the uncertainty. They stated that their questions were always answered but expressed frustration and sometimes anger at always having to initiate the information exchange. There was a sense that the relative was marginalised. A need was expressed for regular information which was routinely volunteered.

Being involved with care

When asked what being involved meant to them, nearly all participants said it meant 'being there' in order to give practical or emotional support to the patient. The practical support consisted of keeping the patient occupied by talking to them, running errands, or helping with language difficulties. The emotional support included reassurance of their continued concern, providing something to look forward to, and trying to alleviate emotional distress.

Almost all felt that being involved with care was a good idea, for the reasons already mentioned but also because it would help the nurses whom they described as being very busy. Reasons for limitations to the amount of involvement possible were given as the age and health of the relative, whether employed or not, and a strong dislike of hospitals. Some suggested that professionals might not like the relatives to be involved as it was their job to care for the patient. Others said that they should leave it to the professionals as they would just get in the way of an already overworked and stretched group.

Relatives' experiences of being involved can be divided into four types: patient generated, relative generated, system generated and professional generated involvement. These are not mutually exclusive.

Patient generated involvement

This occurs because patients want their relatives to be there. Patients are embarrassed about strangers helping them with intimate activities and prefer relatives to assist instead. As one woman said:

> he doesn't like what's happening to him, he's never been in hospital before. So a strong person who does everything for himself and all of a sudden finds himself in that position doesn't want them to touch him, so I think me going there to do it for him makes him feel better.

This situation seems to occur predominantly with male patients who want their wives present, with patients who cannot speak English and with those who have communication problems resulting from a stroke.

Relative generated involvement

This form of involvement occurs because being with the patient helps the relative cope with their anxieties about the situation. Separation from the patient seems to increase these. There is often a need to be with the patient for as long as possible. As one man said: 'I think I was an extreme case because I had to be with him all the time just to make sure he was OK . . . I also think that by being there it gave me more strength, to see that he was recovering and, you know, just reassure myself to be there.' Some also saw it as a way of preparing themselves for when the patient came home.

System generated involvement

Many relatives perceived the health care systems as being overstretched and unable to fulfil all the patients's needs. These relatives seemed to monitor and assess care given and identified gaps in care which they felt they had to fill. These were often related to intimate functions, the time taken to respond to these, or the failure of the nurses to meet these needs thus causing great distress to the patient.

Identifying these gaps provoked different responses from the relatives which were mediated by the nurses' reactions to their subsequent behaviour. Some felt that realistically they could not expect nurses to be with their relative continuously in order to meet all needs, however, others perceived this failure to be due to understaffing and underfunding.

Professional generated involvement

This was the least frequently mentioned category of all. Some relatives had been shown exercises by physiotherapists and placed much importance on encouraging the patient to carry these out regularly, as this was seen as a way of improving the patient's physical problems. No relative mentioned care plans. There were incidences of nurses suggesting that relatives' presence was important for the patients' emotional well-being, and giving ideas of how they might help, e.g. massaging limbs or helping with meals. The main approach seems to be summed up by a woman who said:

lets put it like this, nobody has said anything. Maybe it might not be a bad idea if they do say to relatives, if you want to you can. I mean, I've just done it. I haven't asked is it all right or am I doing wrong. They'd soon tell me. The fact that they've said nothing must mean they're either pleased or they hadn't thought much about it. The sister there is a very nice lady and she's never intimated that anything I've done has been against hospital routine or frowned upon, or anything like that.

It is clear that preferences for being informed and being involved in care are varied and individualistic. It would seem that relatives information needs are generally not being met, although there is confusion about what it is they want to know, leading to an uncertainty about what questions to ask. Relatives may need help to identify and communicate their information needs.

These findings concur with those of Anderson (1992) that the involvement in rehabilitation by the supporters of stroke patients seems to be slight. What involvement that does occur seems to be motivated by the desire to fulfil the patient's needs which are not being met by the health care system. Involvement in care is something that many relatives wish to do. Whether one sees this as an untapped resource or as a method of self-empowerment, there is a need to investigate further ways in which this can be incorporated within hospital settings and specifically within rehabilitation units.

Acknowledgement

I would like to thank the Department of Health for its continued support for this research.

References

Anderson, R. (1992). *The aftermath of stroke: the experience of patients and their families*. Cambridge University Press: Cambridge.

Brownlea, A. (1987). Participation: myths, realities and prognosis. *Social Science and Medicine, 14D*, 139–46.

Greveson, G. C., Gray, C. S. and French, J. M. (1991). Long-term outcome for patients and carers following hospital admission for stroke. *Age and Ageing, 20*, 337–44.

Waterworth, S. and Luker, K. (1990). Reluctant Collaborators: do patients want to be involved in decisions concerning care? *Journal of Advanced Nursing, 15*, 971–6.

13 Client participation in health promotion encounters with health visitors

Sally Kendall

Introduction

The recent White Paper entitled *The Health of the Nation* (Department of Health, 1992) is a (belated) response to the World Health Organisation (1978) call for health for all by the year 2000. It contains five key areas in which health targets are to be achieved in England within the next decade. These include reductions in coronary heart disease and strokes, reductions in mental illness, cancers, accidents and HIV/AIDS. Whilst the document has been criticised for its apparent failure to address the main determinants of ill health such as poverty and for its emphasis on the prevention of illness rather than the promotion of positive health, it does nevertheless provide the first real commitment from the government in supporting the value of health promotion. Importantly for nurses, the document does stress the strategic role that nurses can potentially play in achieving the targets, especially those working in primary health care. This will become all the more significant as the Community Care Act (Department of Health, 1990) takes effect. However, *The Health of the Nation* does not address how health professionals should be engaged in achieving the targets. It would appear that in order to have any positive effect on the five areas mentioned methods of health promotion must be well planned and supported by research and evaluation. Many approaches have been advocated, usefully drawn together and critically discussed by Tones *et al.* (1990). The view taken by the author, supported by others such as Tones (1991), is that to be effective we have to work in partnership with patients and clients and that to do this we have to take an empowering, participative approach to health promotion.

This chapter will begin by exploring the concept of participation and its relationship to health promotion. It will continue by presenting some findings from a recently completed study which found that participation in the health visiting context was evidently not put into practice, and will finish by briefly suggesting some directions for future research and practice.

The concept of participation

The concept of participation in health is closely allied to concepts such as partnership and empowerment. As such, it implies that an egalitarian relationship should exist between the health promoter and the individual or group whose health is to be promoted. However, as Clayton (1988) has argued, the concept of client participation is both complex and underdeveloped as there is no unified meaning to be found in the literature. It ranges from the concept of patient compliance in treatment regimens (Roter, 1977; Ross, 1988), and involvement in decision-making related to treatment and health behaviour (Brody, 1980; Slimmer and Brown, 1985; Valanis and Rumpler, 1985), to increasing patient satisfaction through negotiation (Eisenthal *et al.*, 1983; Greenfield *et al.*, 1985; Littlefield and Adams, 1987) and increasing self-help and self-care at a community level (Drennan, 1985; Brownlea, 1987). All these interpretations of participation may have relevance to nurses at different stages in their relationships with individuals and communities. Even the idea of patient compliance, whilst apparently at odds with the prevailing ideology in health promotion, may have relevance in today's climate of measuring effectiveness through health outcomes such as immunisation uptake, for example. Whilst it has been argued that some clients prefer not to take an active role in their health care (Waterworth and Luker, 1990, for example), in general, the studies cited have shown that people can benefit from participation in health by increasing their autonomy and control.

The importance of client participation was brought to the fore for primary health care nurses by the World Health Organisation (1978) claim: 'The people have the right and duty to participate individually and collectively in the planning and implementation of their health care.' This notion has been reiterated and promoted by subsequent documents and is embodied in the principles for health visiting by the paragraph: 'The facilitation of health enhancing activities' (CETHV, 1977). This suggests that health visitors should take an enabling approach to care, facilitating people to make choices which are right for them, but in so doing providing them with information about health which will help them in their decision-making. This, as Katon and Kleinman (1980) have suggested, would necessitate understanding the clients' view of things, how they explain their health and how they make sense of health promoting activities. This may involve sharing the professional perspective with the client and reaching mutual understanding through recognition of each others beliefs and values.

In 1988, the Health Visitor's Association (HVA) produced a document which promoted the concept of client participation and suggested the way forward for health visiting: 'Health visitors and school nurses must actively pursue the breaking down of barriers in professional/ client relationships and act as facilitators to enable clients to participate in their own health care' (ibid., p. 27). However, the majority of the research on client participation has previously been conducted at the physician–patient level and it was felt to be important for the purposes of the study to be discussed to reach an operational definition of participation which reflected the health promotion function of health visitors.

Whilst the studies on community involvement are clearly relevant to health visitors, it was assumed that, in reality, the majority of health visitors are working at the one-to-one level. Therefore, D'Onofrio's (1980) definition was seen to be helpful in understanding client participation in health visiting. She sees participation as: 'Client involvement in problem identification and prioritisation, establishment of change objectives and the process of making decisions about how change will be accomplished' (ibid., 274).

It seems reasonable in health promotion terms within dyadic relationships that clients should be involved in deciding what their health needs are, what is most important to them, what changes they may need to make and how that change will be achieved. The definition also allows for analysis of participation within the *interaction* between health visitor and client which, as Greenfield *et al.* (1985) point out, is the point at which people currently have the greatest opportunity to participate.

In the light of the current literature on client participation and the prevailing political ideology which claims to promote consumer choice (Department of Health, 1990), it appears that health visitors should be engaging in this approach to practice. The aim of this study was to explore the extent to which client participation was, in fact, a feature of health visiting practice.

Method

A largely qualitative approach was taken to exploring the phenomenon of client participation in health promotion in the health visiting context and therefore a convenience sample of fifteen health visitors was selected for the study. The health visitors ranged in age from 28 to 58 years and had been qualified between 8 weeks and 30 years. Each health visitor was asked to arrange visits to five families with at least one child under one year (excluding primary visits), which were tape recorded, and to participate in an interview following the visit which elicited their perceptions of that visit. The clients were also interviewed shortly after the visit to establish their perceptions of it. Assurances of confidentiality were given to both health visitors and clients and their written consent to be involved in the study obtained. As found by previous researchers in this field (Macleod Clark, 1982; Sefi, 1985; Montgomery Robinson 1987), the use of tape recorders was not found to interfere with the flow of conversation between the health visitors and their clients. A total of sixty-two interactions were successfully recorded and seventy-five pairs of interviews completed. The interactions were transcribed verbatim and analysed using a modified approach to conversation analysis (Heritage, 1984). Whilst it is acknowledged that these interactions only provided a 'snapshot' of practice within a potentially long-term relationship, they nevertheless provided a rich and interesting source of data.

Findings

The overall findings indicate that there is little evidence of either clients initiating an active stance or health visitors promoting client participation.

The interview data, which are not presented here, revealed significant incongruence between health visitors' and clients' perceptions of their health needs. One explanation for this may be found in the way in which interactions were managed. The transcripts were analysed using a modified approach to conversation analysis (Heritage, 1984). Essentially, conversation analysis is concerned with describing the procedures and expectations in terms of which speakers produce their own behaviour and interpret the behaviour of others. Heritage (1984) has suggested that the most fundamental assumption of conversation analysis is that 'all aspects of social action and interaction can be found to exhibit organised patterns of stable, identifiable, structured features,' (ibid., p. 274).

Speakers bring to the conversation knowledge of these organisations which influences their own behaviour and their interpretation of the behaviour of others. Conversation can therefore be analysed to exhibit these organised patterns of action which underlie social activity. In this study it was found that interactions between health visitors and clients had clearly identifiable structures which, overall, led to the conclusion that health visitors were in control of the conversations. For example, it was found that the health visitors set the agenda for the visit, controlled 'turn taking' by asking many questions, gave unsolicited advice and managed closure of a conversation. To illustrate these assertions, some patterns identified in the process of information gathering will be presented.

Gathering and providing information

For the purpose of the analysis of this aspect of the interaction, the collection and provision of information during a home visit was identified as any sequence in which the health visitor attempted to find out about family health needs, problems or resources, or any sequence in which the client articulated her perception of the health needs of the family or the individual; either in response to the health visitor or initiated by herself. Eliciting and understanding the health needs of the family as perceived by the client is clearly essential to the negotiation of any health promotion action which the family decide to take.

To this extent, one could expect to find evidence of health visitors eliciting the health beliefs of the client and trying to understand and share the client's ideas about the health of the family. However, in this study it was found that sharing of ideas was rare and that identified health needs were largely based on the health visitor's agenda. Thus health needs as the clients perceived them could not readily be addressed.

Several approaches were taken by health visitors to the process of information gathering. They included question and answer sequences, where the health visitor asked the questions, question and answer sequences with commentary and observation by the health visitor followed by commentary from the client. Rarely, the sequence would be opened by the client asking a question.

The question and answer sequence

One approach to information gathering was the question and answer sequence. In this technique the health visitor asked the client a direct question about a specific topic to which the client responded. The health visitor then had a choice of two pathways – either to go on to the next question or to respond to the client's answer with a comment, some information or some advice. The nature of the paired sequence of question and answer made it almost impossible for the clients to respond in any other way than to answer the question. It was unusual, for example, for the client to respond with another question or to change the topic. This type of sequence was more likely to occur towards the beginning of an encounter when the health visitor appeared to be gathering a data base of information from which selected needs as perceived by the health visitor could be dealt with later in the interaction.

There are numerous examples of the question and answer sequence since all the interactions include at least one example of it. The following example is typical of sequences where the health visitor elected to move on to the next question:

Line 7 HV   Yes. She's sleeping through the night now?
Line 8 c   Oh yes. She goes down at about nine and I don't hear
             her until about seven . . .
Line 10 HV Uh – uh
Line 11 c   . . . in the morning.
Line 12 HV And we've started on tastes and things like that?
Line 13 c   Oh yes. She's on, um, solids now. She's um, I started her
             this morning actually with a bit of breakfast (Uh – uh) so
             she's having three (Yes) three a day now.
Line 19 HV And you'll soon be cutting out a feed now, won't you?
Line 20 c   Oh yes.

In this sequence the health visitor chose to continue with her questions attempting to gather data rather than respond to the client. However, it is the way in which the questions are posed which is interesting. Whilst collecting her information the health visitor appears to be seeking affirmative responses, thus exposing her own expectations of the child and closing any opportunities the client may need to give negative responses. Indeed, the client may feel it is not acceptable to respond negatively. This is particularly obvious at line 19 where by adding 'won't you' to the end of the question the health visitor in fact leads the client into a positive response. There is no further exploration of this issue or 'cutting out a feed' except that at line 21 the health visitor tells the client it will be 'the lunch time one'. The style comes across as being almost interrogative but is not unusual in the data as a further example demonstrates:

Line 31 HV So what's he doing with his eating? How's he doing with
             his food?
Line 32 c   Oh all right really, on the whole, aren't you? Well, he's
             on three meals a day still and er . . .
Line 34 HV Yes, and does he have a pudding as well as a savoury at
             this time?
Line 35 c   Yes, and a drink of fruit juice.
Line 30 HV And juice. So what about breast feeds now, what are you
             doing?

In this sequence the style remained interrogative by the apparent bombardment of multiple questions, but the questions themselves are more open than in the first example.

The question arises, what are the health visitors doing with all the information they are accumulating in this way? Are they using it to formulate health objectives with the client or are they simply storing the information for its own sake, possibly as a way of maintaining some control over the family's health behaviour? Further analysis of sequences illustrates how this question and answer sequence serves to provide the health visitor with a 'database' of information from which she can select matters which she perceives to have particular relevance or concern to the client.

For example, HVX6B is assessing the nutritional intake of the infant:

Line 60 HV Right, and what are you giving? All tinned food, packet food?
Line 61 C Packet it is. Robinsons.
Line 62 HV Robinsons.
Line 63 C Packet stuff it is (right). Three spoonfuls of dry powder to three of water.
Line 64 HV And that's all the feeds are that, are they?
Line 65 C Yes.
Line 66 HV Right, how's he taken to that?
Line 67 C He seems all right apart from he's a bit loose at the other end. Um, whether thats because of the food or he's just not used to it yet.
Line 69 HV Tell me, when did you change over? Last week?
Line 70 C Yeah, er, it must have been Thursday morning, Wednesday last thing, one day last before I took him up the clinic anyway.
Line 72 HV Right. And has he been sick on his food?
Line 73 C Um, not as much but he is still being sick.

Here, the health visitor appears to be asking a series of questions, building up a bank of information about the baby's diet. The nature of the questioning at lines 60, 64, 66, 69 and 72 would suggest that the health visitor is organising the information in order to give the client some information or advice, but instead she moves on to analysing the consistency of the food: HV Line 89: . . . just tell me, is it Boots, is it very smooth stuff or has it got little lumps in it? It is not until line 123 that the health visitor returns to the baby's loose stools, an issue which was inferred by the client at line 68 as being a problem:

Line 123 HV Right, now, you're saying that his stools are loose now.
Line 124 C Mm. Very loose it is.

The significance of this sequence is that the conversation assumes a question and answer pattern, largely controlled by the health visitor's desire for information and which achieves very little. Indeed, the same point may have been reached similarly by asking the client if she was having any problems with the child's diet. The client cannot be described as participating in this sequence because she has no control over the content or the topic of the questions. The client cannot introduce her own topic with any immediate impact because sequential implicativeness would suggest that questions are responded to and the health visitor does not yield control of the topic to the client. When the client did attempt to introduce her own perceived needs as at line 67, these were overlooked. The value of asking one meaningful question which relates to the client's perceived needs can be seen from a further example:

Line 29 HV What happened about the breast feeding? You rang me up didn't you?

Line 30 C I was going to talk to you about that actually. I'm going to put her on the bottle, I think. I've survived till now but I'm just not doing enough. I eat all the time, but she's hungry all the time. I was doing a top-up feed in the evenings but I'm having to do one at lunch time as well now, 'cos as the day goes on she's getting hungrier and hungrier, I've noticed.

Line 35 HV Right. Are you not comfortable breast feeding?

Whilst this sequence ends in another question, the primary question is more open than in previous examples and has allowed the client to introduce the issues that are troubling her. In this case, the fact that the baby seems hungry despite top-up feeds and the mother's diet being adequate. Even so, by asking another question the health visitor loses the opportunity to allow the client to express and explore ways of meeting her needs, since the health visitor has effectively blocked the interaction with her next turn and does not acknowledge until line 100 that the client actually wants to stop breast feeding.

Line 100 HV So you'd rather forget it completely?

Line 101 C Yeah. I'd rather.

In summary, the question and answer sequence as a technique for collecting information may be used simply as an expedient way of building up a database of information or may be used more constructively to collect information which is relevant to the clients' needs. This would appear to depend on the way in which the sequence is initiated and the extent to which health visitors use their next turn as an opportunity for further questioning. Clearly, health visitors do need to have as full a picture as possible of a situation in order to plan an effective health promotion intervention, but these data seem to suggest that more importance was placed on the information *per se* than on its significance for the client. It is therefore difficult to argue that these health visitors took a participative or enabling approach to health promotion.

Discussion and conclusions

A very small portion of the data from this study has been presented to provide some evidence of the distinctly worrying possibility that the health visitors in this study were not promoting client participation. Clearly, we have to confront the possibility that in day to day health promotion practice health visitors may not be using the interaction effectively in terms of enabling clients to participate.

Whilst one must exercise some caution in generalising from a relatively small study, the findings suggest that the health visitors did not promote client participation and that clients did not take an active part in the interaction. Some of the findings confirm what others have found in studies of health visitor–client interactions during primary visits (Sefi, 1985; Montgomery Robinson, 1987) and also substantiates Pearson's (1991) findings that lay and professional perceptions of health needs may differ. It was not possible for the purposes of this study to follow up the clients at any time after the initial observations, but it would have been interesting to ascertain the extent to which these interactions affect health behaviour. One may speculate, for example, that individuals would be unlikely to act on a health agenda which was not explicitly seeking their perceptions of the health needs of the family.

The question inevitably arises, why is health promotion being practised in this way? The controlling aspect of the health visitors' practice gives rise for concern. It could be that health visitors are acting as agents of social control (Zola, 1972) in order to maintain professional recognition in an era when the future of health visiting hangs in the balance. However, previous research has shown that consumers reject an authoritative approach (McIntosh, 1986; Ashley 1987; Foster and Mayall, 1990). It therefore seems more likely that effective visits in terms of health outcomes will be achieved if health visitors positively promote client participation.

Perhaps some explanation may come from the apparent lack of a coherent conceptual framework for practice. It is in this area where it is imperative to look at improving the effectiveness of health promotion. Through the exploration of theoretical approaches to understanding the client's perspective and working in closer partnership, it may be possible to improve effectiveness. This would also suggest that we need to look more closely at integrating theory and practice, which has implications for how theory is learned. Schon (1983), for example, has popularised the concept of the reflective practitioner. It could be that in order to interact effectively with clients, accepting their values and beliefs about health and enabling them to participate meaningfully, health visitors do need to develop their reflective skills. In terms of research, it is important to carry out carefully designed studies which test the validity of theory in practice, particularly in relation to health outcomes.

In the conclusions of the HVA (1988, pp. 41–2) document it is stated: 'To make progress in health promotion in the spheres of drug abuse, smoking and alcohol consumption, dietary habits, etc., it is essential to have compliance of clients and willingness to participate in programmes'. Whilst the use of the term compliance is unfortunate, the underlying sentiment is well intentioned. However, from the evidence presented in this chapter it appears that health visitors need to develop facilitative skills which will elicit and promote client participation. Clients cannot be expected to be actively involved in and comply with health care recommendations if they are not being acknowledged as equals and their own experiences and perspectives being taken into account. This may mean that, as well as addressing communication skills, health visitors need to address their professional values and attitudes. The apparent need to control clients rather than negotiate with them must be confronted and tackled both at the educational and practice levels, if the health promotion role of the health visitor is to have any real value for the consumer and for the health of the nation.

References

Ashley, Y. (1987). Do health visitors really understand women's needs? Unpublished paper presented at the International Primary Health Care Conference, Westminster (September).

Brody, D. S. (1980). The patient's role in clinical decision making. *Annals of Internal Medicine*, 93, 718–22.

Brownlea, A. (1987). Participation: myths, reality and prognosis. *Social Science and Medicine*, 25, 6, 605–14.

Cassileth, B. *et. al.* (1980). Information and participation preferences among cancer patients. *Annals of Internal Medicine*, 92, 832–6.

Clayton, S. (1988). Patient participation: an undeveloped concept. *Journal of the Royal Society of Health*, 2, 55–8.

Council for Education and Training of Health Visitors (1977). *An Investigation into the Principles of Health Visiting*. CETHV: London.

D'Onofrio, C. N. (1980). Patient compliance and patient education – some fundamental issues, in Squyres, W. (ed.). *Patient Education*. Springer: New York.

Dennis, K. (1987). Dimensions of client control. *Nursing Research*, 36, 3, 151–6.

Department of Health (1990). *NHS and Community Care Act*. HMSO: London.

Department of Health (1992). *The Health of the Nation*. London: HMSO.

Drennan, V. (1985). *Working in a Different Way*. North Paddington District Health Authority: London.

Eisenthal, S., Koopman, C. and Lazare A. (1983). Process analysis of two dimensions of the negotiated approach in relation to satisfaction in the initial interview. *Journal of Nervous and Mental Disease, 171*, 1, 49–54.

Foster, M. C. and Mayall, B. (1990). Health Visitors as educators. *Journal of Advanced Nursing, 15*, 286–92.

Greenfield, S., Kaplan, S. and Ware, J. (1985). Expanding patient involvement in care. *Annals of Internal Medicine, 102*, 520–8.

Haugh, M. R. and Lavin, B. (1979). Public challenge of physician authority. *Medical Care, 17* (8), 844–58.

Health Visitors Association (1988). *Bridging the Gap*. HVA: London.

Heritage, J. (1984). *Garfinkel and Ethnomethodology*. Polity Press: Cambridge.

Katon, N. and Kleinman, A. (1980). Doctor–patient negotiation and other social science strategies in patient care, in Eisenberg, L. and Kleinman, A. (eds). *The Relevance of Social Science for Medicine*. Reidel Publishing: New York.

Kim, H. S. (1985). *Patients attitudes regarding collaborative decision making in nursing*. Unpublished paper, University of Rhode Island.

Littlefield, V. and Adams B. (1987). Patient participation in alternative prenatal care: impact on satisfaction and health locus of control. *Research in Nursing and Health, 10*, 139–48.

Macleod Clark, J. (1982). Nurse–patient verbal interactions: a study of conversations on selected surgical wards. Unpublished Ph.D. thesis, London University.

McIntosh, J. (1986). *A Consumer Perspective on the Health Visiting Service*. Social and Paediatric Research Unit, University of Glasgow.

Montgomery Robinson, K. (1987). The social construction of health visiting. Unpublished Ph.D. thesis, Polytechnic of the South Bank, London.

Pearson, P. (1991). Clients' perceptions: the use of case studies in developing theory. *Journal of Advanced Nursing, 16*, 521–8.

Pendelton, L. and House, W. C. (1984). Preferences for treatment approaches in medical care: college students versus diabetic outpatients. *Medical Care, 22*, 7, 644–6.

Ross, F. (1988). Information sharing for patients, nurses and doctors. Evaluation of a drug guide for old people in primary health care, in Johnson R. (ed.). *Recent Advances in Nursing (21): Excellence in Nursing*. Churchill Livingstone: Edinburgh.

Roter, D. (1977). Patient participation in the patient provider interaction – the effect of question asking on the quality of interaction, satisfaction and compliance. *Health Education Monograph, 5*, 4, 281–315.

Schon, D. (1983). *The Reflective Practitioner*. Englewood Cliffs, NJ: Jossey Bass.

Sefi, S. (1985). The first visit: a study of health visitor/mother verbal interaction. Unpublished M. A. dissertation, University of Warwick.

Slimmer, L. and Brown, R. (1985). Parents' decision making process in medication administration for control of hyperactivity. *Journal of School Health, 55*, 6, 221–5.

Strull, W. M., Bernard, L. and Charles, G. (1984). Do patients want to participate in medical decision making? *Journal of the American Medical Association, 252*, 21, 2990–4.

Tones, K., Tilford, S. and Robinson, Y. (1990). *Health Education – Effectiveness and Efficiency*. Chapman & Hall: London.

Tones, K. (1991). Health promotion, empowerment and the psychology of control. *Journal of the Institute of Health Education, 29*, 1, 17–26.

Valanis, B. G. and Rumpler, C. H. (1985). Helping women to choose breast cancer treatment alternatives. *Cancer Nursing, 8,* 3, 167–75.

Waterworth, S. and Luker, K. (1990). Reluctant collaboraters: do patients want to be involved in decisions concerning care? *Journal of Advanced Nursing, 15,* 971–6.

World Health Organisation (1978). *Alma-Ata, Primary Health Care.* WHO: Geneva.

Zola, I. (1972). Medicine as an institution of social control. *Sociological Review, 20,* 4, 487–509.

14 Practice nursing and health promotion: a case study

Martin Bradford and Sandra Winn

Introduction

The volume of work undertaken in general practice has increased considerably as a result of the 1990 GP contract (Fry, 1991; Hannay *et al.*, 1992). Many of the requirements of the new contract involve health promotion, including health checks and health promotion clinics. In addition to these new services, greater emphasis has been placed upon pre-existing health promotion activities such as cervical cytology screening and immunisation. Much of this health promotion work is carried out by practice staff other than GPs, in particular by practice nurses (Fry, 1991; Stilwell, 1991).

The term practice nurse is used to describe those nurses who are directly employed by GPs, in contrast to community nurses, who are also members of the primary health care team but are employed by health authorities (Greenfield *et al.*, 1987). A further distinction between practice nurses and community nurses is that most of the work of the practice nurse tends to be undertaken in the surgery, while much of the work of community nurses is done in patients' homes. The role of the practice nurse is diverse, and a recent study has shown that practice nurses carry out a wide range of tasks, including clinical procedures such as suture removal and applying dressings, screening and preventive work such as blood pressure monitoring and cervical smears, as well as administrative duties (ibid.). The existence of practice nurses was first acknowledged by the Department of Health in the mid-1970s, and during the 1980s the number of practice nurses expanded rapidly (Robinson, 1990).

The way in which health promotion activities are delivered in general practice is likely to be affected by the attitudes and values of the providers, of whom practice nurses are a key group. The attitudes and values of health promotion providers will in turn be influenced by a multitude of factors including peer groups, psychological and sociological theories encountered during professional training, as well as personal and political philosophies (Muntz, 1988). Thus the

119

attitudes and values of practice nurses, who have a central role in the provision of health promotion, may affect the nature of the health promotion in general practice.

Health promotion strategies employed by health professionals differ according to varying definitions of health (Bechoffer, 1989). Ewles and Simnet (1988) have outlined five models on which health can be promoted ranging from a conservative medical approach to social change, a more radical method. Other models include: the client directed approach, in which action is centred on the clients' stated needs; the behaviour change model which encourages a healthy individual lifestyle; and the educational model which aims to increase the understanding of health issues. Although these models are not separate entities and it is recognised that overlap occurs, they provide a useful tool with which to investigate the preferences of health professionals in the way that they promote health.

This chapter examines the nature of the work carried out by practice nurses in one health district, and using the models outlined above, investigates practice nurses' views about health promotion.

Research methods

A questionnaire was sent to all practice nurses in the Brighton Health District asking for three types of information. First, basic data about the characteristics of practice nurses was elicited (age, sex, qualifications, training, number of years in practice nursing). Second, the nature of the health promotion work undertaken by practice nurses was investigated. Following on from this, practice nurses' views about health promotion were explored by asking respondents to rank in order of personal preference five models of promoting health (medical, client-directed, educational, behaviour change and social change), and to select the model which best described their working practice. Respondents were then given four short statements about the nature of health promotion with which they were asked to agree or disagree using Likert response scales.

The FHSA Practice Nurse Adviser was consulted about the content of the questionnaire, which was amended to take account of her comments. Piloting of the questionnaire could not be undertaken without 'using up' some of the survey population, but the section of the questionnaire designed to obtain views about health promotion had already been tested and proved reliable in previous research (Bradford, 1990), most of the remainder of the questionnaire being concerned with factual information which did not necessitate rigorous piloting. Prior to distribution of the questionnaire, an invitation to give a presentation about the research at the Brighton Practice Nurse

Forum was accepted. This provided an opportunity to encourage the practice nurses present (n = 35) to complete and return the questionnaire. A full database of practice nurse details is held by the FHSA, and this enabled questionnaires to be sent out with a reply paid envelope direct to practice addresses. The response rate was 63 per cent (65 responses from a population of 103). A total of 80 per cent of practices which employ a practice nurse was represented in the sample.

Results

Sample characteristics

Sixty-four of the sixty-five respondents were women. The age distribution, practice nursing experience and qualifications of the sample are shown in *Table 14.1*. The characteristics of the Brighton sample are broadly similar to those of the practice nurses in a 1987 survey undertaken by Greenfield *et al.* in the West Midlands. However, a much larger proportion of the present sample was aged under 30 (16 per cent, compared with 7 per cent in the 1987 survey), and a larger proportion in the present survey had a health visiting qualification (14 per cent, compared with 3 per cent in the 1987 survey). The balance between RGN (92 per cent) and SEN (10 per cent) qualified practice nurses is similar to those recorded in other surveys (Selby, 1992).

The majority of respondents had entered practice nursing relatively recently. This is in accordance with national data trends (DHS, 1990; Stilwell, 1991) and corresponds with the increased GP workload ensuing from the 1990 contract. Practice nursing in this district is a predominantly part-time profession with 67 per cent of respondents indicating that they were employed on this basis. Eighty-nine per cent of respondents worked in a group practice and of those practices with five or more GPs, 75 per cent employed three or more practice nurses.

Current responsibilities of practice nurses

High levels of activity were reported for clinical tasks such as collecting samples, suture removal and immunisations (*Table 14.2*). Although the new contract lays great emphasis on the performance of health promotion duties, the results show that much of the practice nurses' time is devoted to treatment-oriented services. The new duties specified in the 1990 contract, such as health promotion clinics, new registration checks and health checks on the elderly, were carried out by the majority of respondents. In terms of health promotion clinics, diabetes and asthma were the two clinics in which the largest numbers of practice nurses participated (*Table 14.3*). A slightly lower proportion

Table 14.1 *Sample characteristics*

Age distribution	Percentage of respondents (n = 65)	
Under 30	16	
30–39	31	
40–49	25	
50–59	28	

Practice nurse experience (percentages)	Years in practice nursing (n = 65)	Years in present post (n = 65)
Less than 1 year	25	28
1–4 years	39	43
5–10 years	25	17
More than 10 years	12	12

Qualifications	Percentage of respondents (n = 63)	
RGN/SRN	92	
District Nursing Certificate	25	
Health Visiting Diploma	14	
SEN	10	

of practice nurses in the present sample than in Greenfield *et al.*'s 1987 survey reported undertaking specific clinical duties. For example, suture removal was performed by 85 per cent of the present sample compared with 95 per cent of the 1987 sample. In contrast, similar proportions of respondents in both surveys were undertaking those health promotion duties which were carried out in general practice before the introduction of the new contract. Thus 91 per cent of the present sample compared with 95 per cent of the 1987 sample performed immunisations, and 77 per cent of the present sample compared with 71 per cent of the 1987 sample undertook cervical cytology screening.

Respondents were asked whether they contributed to practice meetings, and 70 per cent reported that they did so. The number of years that practice nurses had spent in the professions was proportionally linked to contributing at practice meetings, with 75 per cent of those who had spent more than ten years in the profession contributing at

Table 14.2 *Current responsibilities of respondents*

	Percentage of respondents (n = 65)
Immunisations	91
Health promotion clinics	88
Sutures	85
Collecting samples	83
Cervical cytology screening	77
Administration	74
Health checks on elderly people	71
New registration checks	69
Counselling/advice	51
Minor surgery	51
Family planning	39
Health checks on non-attenders	32
Ante-natal clinics	20
Health checks on children	14

Table 14.3 *Health promotion clinics undertaken by respondents*

	Percentage of all clinics (n = 163)
Diabetes	17
Asthma	15
Weight control	13
Well woman	13
Well person	11
Well man	5
Hypertension	5
Other[1]	21

[1] Other includes smoking, coronary heart disease, travel immunisation.

practice meetings, compared with 62 per cent of those who had been in practice nursing for less than a year.

Seventy-five per cent of practice nurses said they would like more health promotion or clinical training. There were no statistically significant differences between age groups or between practice nurses

Table 14.4 *Training needs identified by respondents (n = 45)*

Health issue	Percentage of all training needs
Family planning	17%
Counselling	14%
Well woman	11%
Cervical cytology	9%
General update	9%
Other[1]	40%

[1] Other includes ear syringing, asthma, diabetes, HIV/AIDS.

with different professional qualifications in terms of the proportion of respondents who said they would like further training. *Table 14.4* shows that the training needs of respondents are predominantly in areas of health promotion rather than clinical.

Views about health promotion

Respondents were asked to rank five models of promoting health and to indicate which one they used in practice (*Table 14.5*). Two of the more radical health promoting models, the social change and educational models, together were ranked highest by 58 per cent of respondents. However, the pattern of support for these models is complex (*Figure 14.1*). For the social change model of promoting health respondents' views were polarised. Although 22 per cent of respondents rated the social change model highest, it was also ranked lowest by 64 per cent. One factor contributing to this polarised response may be respondents' use of the social change model in practice, because only one respondent indicated that she did so. Conversely, the medical model was ranked highest by only 9 per cent of respondents, but was reported to be the model used in practice by 37 per cent of respondents (*Figure 14.2*). The behaviour change model, which reflects a prescriptive approach to promoting health, was ranked highest or second highest by 50 per cent of respondents, while the client-directed model was only ranked highest by 13 per cent of respondents.

Younger practice nurses were more likely to support the radical models of promoting health. Twenty-nine per cent of the under 40 age group and 15 per cent of the over 40 group ranked the social change model of promoting health highest. The under 30 age group compared with all other age groups provided a starker differential with 43 per

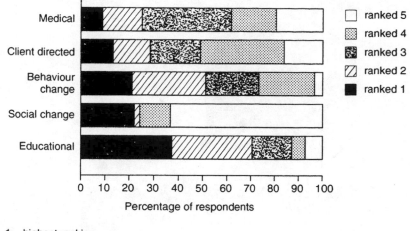

1 = highest ranking
5 = lowest ranking

Figure 14.1 *Rankings of models*

Table 14.5 *Rankings of models of promoting health*

	Percentage of respondents ranking model highest	Percentage of respondents ranking model lowest	
Educational[1]	36	8	(n = 50)
Social change[2]	22	64	(n = 50)
Behaviour change[3]	22	2	(n = 46)
Client directed[4]	13	17	(n = 47)
Medical[5]	9	20	(n = 46)

[1] 'Promoting an understanding of health issues enabling patients to make an informed choice.'
[2] 'Working to change political and social environments to make healthier choices easier choices.'
[3] 'Encouraging people to change to healthier lifestyles.'
[4] 'Working on health issues identified by the client.'
[5] 'Promoting medical intervention through persuasive methods, screening, vaccination etc.'

cent of the under 30 group and 17 per cent of the over 30 group ranking the social change model highest, although the difference is not statistically significant (Fisher's exact test, $p > 0.05$). The support of younger age groups for more radical models is underlined by the resistance of these groups to the most conservative model, the medical model. A total of 25 per cent of respondents aged under 40 rated the medical model lowest, compared with only 17 per cent of respondents aged over 40.

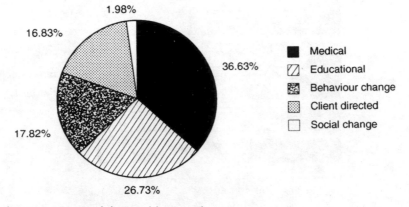

Figure 14.2 *Models used in practice*

Table 14.6 *Association between rankings of models and contribution to practice meetings*

Model ranked highest	Percentage of respondents contributing at practice meetings (n = 49)
Social change	91
Educational model	61
Client directed	100
Behaviour change	60
Medical	25

Those respondents who ranked the social change or client-directed models highest were most likely to contribute at practice meetings, while those who ranked the medical model highest were least likely to contribue (*Table 14.6*). Comparing respondents who rated the medical or behaviour change models highest with those who did not, the difference in participation at practice meetings is not statistically significant at the 0.05 level (χ^2 = 3.468 with 1 d.f., p < 0.10).

There was little relationship between the number of years that respondents had spent in practice nursing and the rankings of the models of health promotion. Twenty-one per cent of respondents who had been in the profession for less than five years ranked the social change model highest, compared with 20 per cent of those who had more than five years practice nursing experience. Similar results were obtained for the other models, and these findings were replicated when the number of years in present post was analysed by rankings of models. Respondents also gave similar rankings of models regardless of professional qualification, and the model used in practice did not differ between qualification groups.

Using Likert response scales, respondents were asked to indicate the extent to which they agreed or disagreed with statements about the nature of health promotion (*Table 14.7*). Statements (b), (c) and (d) in *Table 14.7* are linked to the most radical model of promoting health, the social change model, while statement (a) reflects the most conservative models, the medical and behaviour change models. Overall, respondents were more in agreement with the radical statements of health promotion and more than half of the respondents disagreed with the most conservative statement. The statement with which the largest proportion of respondents were in agreement (88 per cent) is, 'If I spend time educating people about their health they in turn will educate others'. Statement (c), which extends the concept of enablement beyond the individual, produced a slightly lower level of

Table 14.7 *Views about health promotion statements (percentages)*

	Agree or strongly agree	Neutral	Disagree or strongly disagree	
(a) Patients are not concerned with issues beyond their own health status	23	23	54	(n = 65)
(b) If I spend time educating people about their health they in turn will educate others	88	6	6	(n = 65)
(c) Health promotion should enable individuals, families and communities to reach their own decisions about health issues	80	13	8	(n = 64)
(d) Health promotion should include meeting people to work together to change health policy	55	42	3	(n = 65)

agreement (80 per cent), while there was a considerably lower level of agreement (55 per cent) with statement (d), 'Health promotion should include meeting people to work together to change health policy', and a large proportion of respondents (42 per cent) remained neutral to this statement.

A breakdown of responses by age shows some relationship between age and agreement with the more radical statements. Thus, for example, while 93 per cent of respondents aged under 40 agreed that the health information that they give will be passed on, only 81 per cent of respondents aged over 40 agreed with this. The differential is increased when the responses of the under 30 age group are compared with those of the over 50 group, where 100 per cent and 71 per cent respectively agreed that their patients would pass on health information. Similarly, whilst 80 per cent of the under 30 age group disagreed with statement (a), 'Patients are not concerned with issues beyond their own health status', only 35 per cent of the 50–9 age group disagreed. This result is statistically significant (Fisher's Exact Test, $p = 0.009$). Conversely, although almost one half of respondents in the over 50 age group were in agreement with this statement not one respondent in the under 30 group was in agreement. However, the relationship between age and views about health promotion is not a simple one. Eighty-seven per cent of respondents aged over 40 compared with only 70 per cent of respondents aged under 40, agreed with the statement, 'Health promotion should enable individuals, families and communities to reach their own decisions about health issues'. Furthermore, in response to the most radical statement, 'Health promotion should get people together to work for change in health policy', the over 40 and under 40 age groups produced similar results, with 53 per cent and 57 per cent in agreement respectively.

The number of years that respondents had spent in practice nursing had little association with their responses to the health promotion statements. Almost identical responses were recorded for all statements from those who had been in the profession for less than five years and those who had more than five years experience.

Respondents who were in agreement with the more radical statements were found to be those who also ranked the more radical models of promoting health the highest. This demonstrates the consistency and value of these models as an investigative theory for health promotion.

Discussion

Practice nurses undertake a wide range of tasks, and most carry out both treatment-oriented and health promoting work. Thus, most practice nurses in this district are not employed solely to undertake the preventive work set out in the new contract. The high levels of activity reported for clinical tasks are to be expected, since these were well established duties of the practice nurse before the new contract. In terms of the health promotion workload resulting directly from the 1990 contract, the activity which the largest numbers of practice nurses undertake is health promotion clinics. Of these, diabetes and asthma are the two clinics most frequently undertaken by practice nurses. These could be seen as disease management rather than strictly primary health promotion, and despite the existence of FHSA protocols for these clinics their position as primary health promotion clinics is debatable.

Comparison of the results with those of Greenfield *et al.* (1987) provide some evidence that in addition to the new health promotion responsibilities assumed by practice nurses since 1990, there has been a slight shift in the other tasks undertaken, with more emphasis now on health promotion activities rather than treatment-oriented work. Some practice nurses do not have contracts, job descriptions or protocols (Stilwell, 1991), in which case the new emphasis on health promotion work could prove to be important in establishing a stronger role definition for the profession. Indeed, it may be that health promotion will provide an appropriate avenue for and extended role for the practice nurses since there is evidence that the scope for extension into medical areas is less certain (Greenfield *et al.*, 1987).

Given the developing nature of the role and professionalisation of the practice nurse it would seen important for practice nurses to be aware of current developments in their field and to incorporate these into their work. The importance of health promotion training is underlined in this investigation where training needs identified by practice nurses were centred around health promotion issues.

The pattern of views about health promotion among practice nurses is complex. While a majority of practice nurses expressed support for either the social change or the educational model of promoting health, almost two-thirds of respondents ranked the social change model lowest, suggesting a diversity of views within the profession about appropriate health promotion strategies. The high level of support for the educational model is reflected in the extent of agreement with the statement, 'If I spend time educating people about their health they in turn will educate others'. These results suggest that respondents believe that their patients will convey health messages which they themselves have imparted and recognise that the influence of the practice nurse extends beyond the individual. The level of agreement with this statement also suggests that practice nurses perceive themselves as having an educational role and are willing to spend time providing people with health information. The lower level of agreement with the statement 'Health promotion should enable individuals, families and communities to reach their own decisions about health issues' suggests that while educating the individual is widely accepted by practice nurses as a feature of health promotion, the concept of empowering groups is less so. Considerably fewer practice nurses agreed with the statement 'Health promotion should include meeting people to work together to change health policy', and a large proportion expressed a neutral position. The implication of this may be that while many practice nurses recognise that health promotion has socio-political implications, the concept appears to be far removed from their working practice. This relates to the finding that although 22 per cent ranked the social change model highest, only 2 per cent said that it was the model that they used in practice. Thus it seems that there is some agreement in principle with more radical approaches to health promotion, but their application in practice nursing is at present limited.

Further evidence of the interaction between working practice and views about health promotion is provided by the association between contributing to practice meetings and support for the more radical models of promoting health. Those who favour more radical models of promoting health are more likely to view health as the product of a wide range of physical, social, economic and political influences (Ewles *et al.*, 1988). Thus, it may be that those respondents who rank the more radical models highest believe that their participation in these forums can affect health care provision and policy. Conversely, those favouring the more individualistic medical or behaviour change models may be less likely to believe that health can be promoted in these ways, and therefore participate less.

The way in which practice nurses perform health promotion services, that is, the content and structure and context of health promotion clinics and health checks, will strongly influence the nature of health promotion in general practice. The prominence of the use of the medical model of promoting health amongst practice nurses and the types of health promotion clinics undertaken by respondents suggests that health promotion services are at present largely prescriptive and centred upon the individual, rather than providing a wider and social emphasis. Clearly, the attitudes of practice nurses towards health promotion and the factors which may influence these attitudes are key determinants of the way in which health promotion services are provided in general practice. The general empathy of the younger respondents with more radical models and statements of health promotion may be one factor which in the longer term will bring about changes in the nature of health promotion in general practice.

Conclusion

Provision of health promotion services is central to the role of the practice nurse in this district, but practice nurses are also responsible for a wide range of treatment related duties. It could be that the diversity of the workload of practice nurses produces a degree of role conflict for them. Views about health promotion amongst practice nurses are diverse, but it is clear that for many there is a discrepancy between their views about health promotion and their working practice. However, there is also evidence that views about health promotion interact with working practice. Given that younger members of the profession are the most supportive of a radical approach to health promotion, it may be that over the next few years there will be a gradual change in the way in which health promotion services are provided.

As general practice seeks to develop and refine its health promotion role, it would seem complementary that practice nurses should also extend and establish this dimension of their role. Through increased health promotion training of practice nurses the advancement of health promotion, and with it the role of the practice nurse, seems assured in general practice.

References

Bechoffer, F. (1989). Individuals politics and society, in Martin, C. and McQueen, D. (eds). *Readings for a New Public Health.* Edinburgh University Press: Edinburgh.

Bradford, M. (1990). *Health promotion in Brighton: An investigation of attitudes towards the proposed Brighton Healthy Living Centre.* Unpublished dissertation, Department of Community Studies, University of Brighton.

Department of Health (1990). Department of Health statistics for general medical practitioners in England and Wales 1978–1988. *Statistical Bulletin, 4* 6, p. 9.

Ewles, L. and Simnett, I. (1988). *Promoting Health: A Practical Guide to Health Education.* Wiley: Chichester.

Fry, J. (1991). The contract: is it working? *Update*, 15 July, 71–2.

Greenfield, S., Stilwell, B., Drury, M. (1987). Practice nurses: social and occupational characteristics. *Journal of the Royal College of General Practitioners, 37,* 341–5.

Hannay, D., Usherwood, T., Platts, M. (1992). Workload of general practitioners before and after the new contract. *British Medical Journal, 304,* 615–18.

Muntz, A. (1988). Value judgements in health visiting, *Health Visitor, 61,* 145–6.

Robinson, G. (1990). The future for practice nurses, *British Journal of General Practice, 40,* pp. 132–3.

Selby, A. (1992). More practice, *Health Service Journal*, 19 March, 31.

Stilwell, B. (1991). The rise of practice nurse, *Nursing Times, 87,* 26–8.

15 Assessment of older people at home – a missed opportunity?*

Ann C. Pursey and Karen A. Luker

Introduction

The contract for general practitioners (GPs) introduced in April 1990 and the Community Care Act which becomes operational in April 1993 have put the issue of assessment of the needs of older people, people with mental health problems and people with learning disabilities clearly on to the policy agenda. In addition, the last five years have seen a shift in the emphasis of government health care policy from the provision of a 'sickness and treatment' service to one which encapsulates the concepts of health promotion and education.

This chapter describes a section of the findings of a research study undertaken during the period October 1989 to September 1992 which attempted to uncover the roles and responsibilities of health visitors and practice nurses, with regard to the assessment of people aged 75 and over in their own homes.

Practice nursing and the GP contract

In April 1990, a new contract for GPs was introduced and heralded a range of additional responsibilities for general practitioners and their practice staff. The contract encouraged a shift from the 'traditional' role of GPs, which was oriented around illness detection and treatment, to increasing their involvement in health promotion and illness prevention activities. It was stated that 'health promotion and disease prevention fall clearly within the definition of General Medical Services' (Health Departments of Great Britain, 1989) and a whole range of activities

* This study was funded by the Department of Health under the nurse studentship scheme.

aimed at encouraging involvement in these areas was outlined. Amongst the new responsibilities was a requirement for GPs to offer each patient aged over 75 years who was registered with the practice an annual home visit to assess their health and social well-being. The outline within the contract of what the assessment should consist of came under the heading 'health promotion/illness prevention' and was divided into the following eight subheadings:

- to see the home environment and to find out whether carers and relatives are available
- social assessment (lifestyle, relationships)
- mobility assessment (walking, sitting, use of aids)
- mental assessment
- assessment of the senses (hearing and vision)
- assessment of incontinence
- general functional assessment
- review of medication

(Taken from the 1990 contract, Health Departments of Great Britain, 1989.)

The guidelines within the contract were no more explicit as to how these areas should be assessed or what tools might be used, leaving this up to the discretion of individual GPs.

In anticipation of the additional responsibilities of the new contract, there was a massive increase in the number of practice nurses employed by GPs (who received at that time a 70 per cent reimbursement of a practice nurse's salary) to undertake a variety of activities on their behalf within the GP practice. In 1989, the number of full-time equivalent practice nurses employed by GPs was 4898 for England and Wales. By the end of 1990 this number had risen to 8155, an increase of almost 100 per cent (all figures from Department of Health, 1991). This large increase in numbers appeared to be the direct result of the changes in the GP contract, and the fact that Family Health Services Authorities (then called Family Practitioner Committees) actively encouraged GPs to employ practice nurses before April 1990 when new cash limits on employment of staff were imposed (Liverpool FHSA, 1990).

It is clear that many practice nurses employed by GPs are expected to take responsibility for a wide range of health promotion activities within the GP surgery, one of these activities being the assessment of people aged 75 and over in their own homes. The suitability and competence of practice nurses who did not hold a community nursing qualification (either district nursing or health visiting) to undertake this work has been called into question (*Nursing Standard News*, 1990). Nevertheless, many practice nurses did, and continue to, visit older people at home.

Early research studies had identified the role of the practice nurse as diverse and multifunctional but mainly oriented around the carrying out of 'traditional nursing' tasks such as height and weigth measurement and temperature recording (Baldwin, 1967; Marsh, 1967). By 1976, Marsh and Chew (1984) had noted that the role of the practice nurse was beginning to change to include more complex functions such as family planning and women's health screening, and later identified the work of the practice nurse in men's health clinics. More recent research work has shown that practice nurses are involved in performing a wide range of technical tasks (Greenfield *et al.*, 1987: Cater and Hawthorn, 1988) and the variation in the extent and nature of their contribution to the practice workload was noted in a report by the Royal College of Nursing (1984). A study in Oxfordshire demonstrated the increasing involvement of practice nurses in health promotion activities (Fowler *et al.*, 1988) and it was suggested that they may be the nurses 'who will lead the team in the health promotion of the future' (ibid.).

There is some evidence that GPs lack commitment to the identification of needs for prevention in the practice population (Coulter and Schofield, 1991), and it is unclear to what extent the potential for health promotion and illness prevention is being realised. What is clear, however, is that the role of health visitors, who are trained to undertake health promotion activities, has been largely ignored in recent policy documents. It is to this group of health care professionals, and their role in work with older people, that we now turn our attention.

Health visitors

It has been evident for some time that the work of the health visitor is mainly oriented towards the child population (Dingwall, 1977; Luker, 1978; Phillips, 1988), with low priority being given to older people. There is evidence, though, that health visitors can be effective in working with older people Barber, 1984; Luker, 1978; Vetter *et al.*, 1984). A recent study of the attitudes of community nurse and general practitioners towards work with older people showed that health visitors considered that they should have a role, particularly in the area of assessment, and that they believed regular assessment for older people was necessary and important (Tremellen and Jones, 1989).

It is well recognised that the health visitor's role with the older population is underdeveloped and that they are trapped with the 0–5 age group (McClymont *et al.*, 1986; de la Cuesta, 1992). In spite of the professional rhetoric which has attempted to shift the health visiting profession towards increasing its involvement with older people (BGS and HVA, 1986), examination of the national statistics shows that the percentage of older people in contact with the health visiting service has remained fairly small (approximately 11 per cent of health visitors total time being spent with older people) over the last decade (Department of Health, 1991). Nevertheless, on a theoretical level, health visitors are trained to undertake health promotion activities with a wide spectrum of the population, including 'well' older people. However, the evidence is that they provide a reactive, crisis-driven service (de la Cuesta, 1992) and do not, in the main, visit that section of the older population who could be considered to be 'well'.

Background to the study

The research study arose out of personal experience of health visiting which had led us to realise that the majority of health visitors do not undertake health promotion activities with well older people. During the initial stages of the research work, the content of the contract for GPs was announced and it seemed that, whilst health visitors held a *theoretical remit* for this work, the *policy remit* for visiting well older people was being passed to the GP and practice nurses through the requirement for assessment of people aged 75 and over within the contract. The research therefore attempted to uncover the role of these two groups of nurses in assessment and health promotion activities with older people at home.

Methods used in the study

In order to build a broad picture of the research area a multimethod approach to data collection was adopted. Pilot work conducted in the early part of 1990 revealed that health visitors had difficulty talking about their work with older people because of the spasmodic nature of their visits. The study was designed in two phases, the first of which aimed to encourage health visitors and practice nurses to describe specific visits to individual older people.

Phase 1 of the study consisted of a questionnaire containing a mixture of forced-choice and open-ended questions and this was completed by a convenience sample of 49 practice nurses, 62 student health visitors and 25 experienced health visitors (defined as those with two or more years' experience) working in the North-West of England. Whilst the content of the questionnaire for each of the three groups was slightly different, the focus was the same and was broadly oriented around issues concerning current and past work with older people. The questionnaire also incorporated a section where the respondents were asked to describe two incidents where they had been involved with an older person/people: one where they felt they had been particularly 'effective' and one where they felt they had been particularly 'ineffective'. This broadly followed the guidelines of a research tool known as Flanagan's Critical Incident Technique (Flanagan, 1954).

Phase 2 of the study involved a theoretical subsample of the Phase 1 respondents, who were each asked to participate in an in-depth conversational interview. These interviews focused broadly on the structural context of practice nursing and health visiting work and student health visitor training. Eight practice nurses, eight student health visitors (at the end of training) and six experienced health visitors agreed to participate in the interviews, which were tape recorded and lasted between forty-five minutes and two hours.

The data yielded from the questionnaire were analysed statistically with the use of the Statistical Package for the Social Sciences (SPSS-pc +). The critical incident data and interview data were analysed using a thematic content analysis and were organised with the facilities available on the Ethnograph computer package.

Findings

Analysis of the questionnaire data indicated that the overall picture of the practice nurses who participated in this study was that they were employed on a G grade (n = 30; 61 per cent), worked with two or more GPs in the practice (n = 46; 94 per cent) and were employed on a part-time basis (n = 41; 84 per cent). Eight (16 per cent) of the sample of 49 practice nurses held a community nursing qualification (either HV or DN certificates) and 29 (59 per cent) of them were involved on a regular basis in visiting older people at home for the purposes of assessment. They visited an average of 23 people aged 75 and over per month.

The majority of the student health visitor respondents already held a post-basic nursing qualification of some description (n = 50, 81 per cent) and rated work with older people at a lower level of satisfaction than work with children (n = 45; 72 per cent for older people compared with 46; 90 per cent for children). They were also more likely to have worked with children before entering health visiting (n = 49; 80 per cent) than with older people (n = 28; 46 per cent).

The experienced health visitor group typically worked full-time (n = 24; 96 per cent) and visited an average of two people aged 75 and over per month.

In terms of previous experience of working with older people 43 (32 per cent) of the 135 respondents (one non-respondent) had held a

Table 15.1 *Number of respondents in each group with post-basic experience caring for older people*

	Previous job caring for older people	No previous job caring for older people
Practice nurses	13 (26%)	36 (74%)
Experienced health visitors	2 (8%)	23 (92%)
Student health visitors	28 (46%)	33 (54%)
Total	43 (32%)	92 (68%)

post-basic position working with older people. *Table 15.1* shows the distribution of this between the three groups. In general, the findings indicated that respondents were less likely to express satisfaction with work with older people than with work with children.

Approaches to assessment

Analysis of the critical incident and interview data revealed that practice nurses, health visitors and student health visitors visited older people for the purposes of assessment, but that there was a huge variety in both the approach to and structure of the assessments. Many of the practice nurses used a card issued by one of several major drug companies with which to structure their assessments. The health visitors, by comparison, were more likely to use a conversational approach to the assessment and did not, in the main, use guidelines or any sort of structured interview schedule. It was apparent that neither the health visitors nor the practice nurses adhered to any type of model or had any philosophy which underpinned their approach to assessment. The student health visitors revealed their confusion as to what a health visitor assessment of an older person was and what they were supposed to achieve (the goals). It was, however, apparent that the approach to assessment was broadly oriented around the detection of functional deficits and identifying problems. In the case of the practice nurses there was notably a stronger emphasis on the detection of unmet medical need, predictable perhaps when one considers that they are employed by general medical practitioners.

It was clear that neither the practice nurse nor the health visitor groups considered that it was their remit to provide health promotion, education and advice to the well older people they visited. The health visitor visits to older people occurred in response to a referral from another agency and the people they visited were already defined as being 'in need' by that agency. Without exception they did not visit the 'well' older population. When the practice nurses visited well older people (which they all did) their role finished with completing the assessment and then returning the following year to undertake another assessment. With the exception of one practice nurse, they did not use the visit as an opportunity for therapeutic interaction with the older person.

Discussion

None of the respondents in this study saw a role for themselves in providing health promotion, education and advice for the older people they visited. It is not clear why this was, although there was some evidence that the respondents did not value or see the purpose of health promotion work with older people. Indeed, they saw old age as a time of deterioration, increasing dependency and a high likelihood of disability. As a consequence of these powerful beliefs about old age, they did not use the assessment visit as anything more than a means to collect information and to refer people in whom they detected previously unmet needs or functional deficits to other agencies. The chance to provide health education and advice to older people during the visits was not exploited by these nurses and this is described as a 'missed opportunity'.

In conclusion, the wider issue within the nursing profession should perhaps be about the relative merits of a specialist nursing input for older people as opposed to a generalist input, particularly with regard to the provision of health promotion and education. The evidence that student health visitors with previous post-basic experience of working with older people express a higher level of satisfaction with work with older people in general than those with no post-basic experience should perhaps stimulate managers to consider previous experience when employing nurses to work with older people. In addition, the potential for assessment visits to be a forum for the provision of health promotion for older people should be addressed by policy-makers, nurse managers and nurse educationalists alike.

References

Baldwin, J. T. (1967). The use of a nurse in general practice. *Journal of the Royal College of General Practitioners, 13,* 364–7.

Barber, J. H. (1984). Screening and surveillance of the elderly at risk. *Practitioner, 228,* 1389, 269–73.

British Geriatric Society (BGS) and Health Visitors Association (HVA) (1986). *Health visiting for the health of the aged. A joint policy statement.* BGS and HVA: London.

Cater, L. and Hawthorne, P. (1988). A survey of practice nurses in the UK, in Bowling, A. and Stilwell, B, (eds), *The Nurse in Family Practice*. Scutari Press: London.

Coulter, A. and Schofield, T. (1991). Prevention in general practice: the views of doctors in the Oxford region. *British Journal of General Practice, 41*, 4, 140–3.

de la Cuesta, C. (1992). Marketing the service: basic social process in health visiting. Unpublished Ph.D. thesis, University of Liverpool.

Department of Health (1991). *Practice Nurse Workforce Statistics*. HMSO: London.

Dingwall, R. (1977). *The Social Organisation of Health Visitor Training*. Croom Helm: London.

Flanagan, J. C. (1954). The critical incident technique. *Psychological Bulletin, 51*, 327–58.

Fowler, G., Fullard, E. and Muir Gray, J. A. (1988). The extended role of practice nurses in preventive health care, in Bowling, A. and Stilwell, B. (eds). *The Nurse in Family Practice*. Scutari Press: London.

Greenfield, S., Stilwell, B. and Drury, M. (1987). Practice nurses: social and occupational characteristics. *Journal of the Royal College of General Practitioners, 37*, 341–5.

Health Departments of Great Britain (1989). *General practice in the National Health Service: The 1990 Contract*. HMSO: London.

Liverpool Family Health Services Authority (1990). Personal communication.

Luker, K. A. (1978). Goal attainment: a possible model for assessing the role of the health visitor. *Nursing Times, 74*, 30, 1257–9.

Marsh, G. N. (1967). Group practice nurse: an analysis and comment on six months' work. *British Medical Journal, 1*, 489–91.

Marsh, G. N. and Chew, C. (1984). Well man clinic in general practice. *British Medical Journal, 288*, 200–1.

McClymont, M., Thomas, S. and Denham, J. (1986). *Health Visiting and the Elderly*. Churchill Livingstone: London.

Nursing Standard News (1990), 4, 31, 5.

Phillips, S. (1988). Health visitors and the priority of the elderly. *Health Visitor, 61*, 341–2.

Royal College of Nursing (1984). *Training Needs of Practice Nurses. Report of a Steering Group*. RCN: London.

Tremellen, J. and Jones, D. A. (1989). Attitudes and practices of the primary health care team towards assessing the very elderly. *Journal of the Royal College of General Practitioners, 39*, 142–4.

Vetter, N. J., Jones, D. E. and Victor, C. R. (1984). Effect of health visitors working with elderly patients: a randomised controlled trial. *British Medical Journal, 48*, 1, 44–5.

SECTION THREE

Developing the nurse's health promotion role

Asserting individual or group rights is an important component of health promoting activity, especially when these groups are at risk of being overlooked and less able to be fully independent or politically active. Child care is an excellent example and projects from across the seas use principles of full representation and education to empower children. Results show that altered health services may be more user-friendly and more in tune with what is seen as acceptable. Their health status and satisfaction also improves.

However, work by Igoe and others demonstrates that particular groups require not only a different programme of health-promoting measures but also that these need to be delivered in sensitive ways. Abilities to master skills and adjust to changes alter throughout the lifespan. The settings and messages deemed necessary for health care have, to date, rarely been sufficiently welcoming, appealing or familiar in type to special groups. Lessons from such responsive (or non-responsive) organisations and individual practitioners attempting to empower families and children in North America and Finland demonstrate that specific attempts are being made to use health-promoting principles to support self-care through a greater level of health education for children. Interestingly, motivational problems are not manifest among children involved. It seems to be the parents and teachers who need to change perspectives and encourage fuller participation from all involved. Much can be learned from these examples and collaborative networks at multiple levels seem to be fundamental to success.

Changing the model for providing assessment and planned care is seen as necessary for promoting health in several of these following contributions. For instance, the elderly require a broad, more consumer-led service and may not be served well by the medically oriented assessment which so frequently occurs.

More imaginative definitions of 'vulnerability' also seem to emerge. Once more, social context, finances and the responses to ill health by others seem to increase vulnerability. Lack of resources and social support can have rapid effects on health status, both physical and mental. Women are clearly seen as under privileged and dependant in many countries and in certain regions within richer nations, as Renfrew demonstrates. Long-standing cultural mores have determined a subservient and passive role for women in many cultures. They fail to reach their potential as responsible and intelligent people and are frequently discriminated against. Many international agencies are targeting them for support. From education on technical matters, such as mending water taps to child care, the health of many nations may be affected positively if women are helped in these ways. Clearly, child rearing is a vital role and future health patterns may be influenced in early life. Empowerment in this way can be so vital and organisations, such as Save the Children Fund, have established many such programmes. True participation by local people is needed with agencies supporting the infrastructure and negotiating government support. As with most country-wide innovations, promoting health, better agricultural development and water supplies are essential. Birth control, hygiene and condom protection against venereal disease come close seconds in the war against poverty.

Recent work on mental health promotion is also affecting our understanding of holistic care and of the reasons why this is important. The value of providing comprehensive care that recognises the interaction of physical with psychological and social factors has been reinforced by much professional literature and by this book. Those with physical problems tend to have negative emotional reactions, many of which may be detrimental to recovery or adjustment. Likewise those with poor mental health and prolonged stress may be far more vulnerable to poor physical health. Promoting mental health by meaningful support, by facilitating awareness of problems and through encouraging positive support is fundamental to the work of many professionals. Nurses in particular are in a position to recognise signs of mental distress and those at risk and should have the general support skills needed to assist those who are troubled, thus preventing possible illness.

Several of the following contributions also point to the need for peer-group support among staff to prevent ill health. Nurses have been shown to be greatly at risk of mental illness, such as stress responses and burn-out (Skevington, 1988). Lack of peer support and under-standing by management is frequently cited. Of late, as the world recession deepens, health resourcing is reduced in most countries. The effect on staff levels on both community teams and hospital establishments is obvious. This, combined with pressure to increase 'turnover' of patients, really raises the level of acute care needed. Dissatisfaction with the quality of comprehensive care given by nurses themselves adds to the stress of the situation.

Successful groups working under strain devise ways in which individuals feel supported and valued. Rewards and appreciation need to be built into the system to maintain morale and prevent illness. Organisational health policies are discussed later by Adams, but it is imperative that managers realise efficiency is based on good morale and team support. Acknowledgement and expressed concern may not be enough, but, without even this, nursing work may become intolerable.

Reference

Skevington, S. (1988). *Occupation Psychology and Nursing*. John Wiley: Chichester.

16 *Healthier children through empowerment*

Judith B. Igoe

Background

Research, pilot demonstrations and innovations in clinical practice offer a foundation for meeting the essential requirements for healthier children under the demands of today's radically altered society. The potential implications of empowering children and families within the health care system in general, and on nursing in particular, are great. This chapter examines how empowerment might improve nursing practice, refine research and enhance the education efforts provided by nurses at home, at school and in the community.

Technology has dramatically improved the potential for healthy children during the twentieth century. Millions of children, who in an earlier age would not have survived to adulthood, are spared through immunisations. Before 1974 only 5 per cent of the world's children received immunisations (Bloom, 1990), but now, the World Health Assembly's goal to immunise 80 per cent of the world's children by 1990 has been met (Nakajima and Grant, 1991).

Advances in technology have fostered changing epidemiological patterns, and in developed countries non-communicable diseases are now the cause of 70–80 per cent of all deaths (WHO, 1991). These non-communicable diseases, predominantly heart disease and cancer in adulthood, are largely attributed to lifetime lifestyle choices, such as smoking, diet and physical activity. Whereas scientific advances have been most effective in reducing the impact of communicable disease, education and counselling are proving to be effective strategies in confronting lifestyle-related health problems.

Education, when properly employed, becomes a process of empowerment, and recent studies have demonstrated how effective education can be in confronting lifestyle-related problems. For example, children with elevated LDL cholesterol were studied at Children's Hospital of Philadelphia. After a ten-week education programme for children combining audio-visual and printed lessons in game form, along with an instructional manual for parents, a significant increase in the children's knowledge of 'heart smart' foods was detected, along with a trend towards reductions of their base-line consumption of total fat, saturated fat, and cholesterol (Shannon *et al.*, 1991). In another study, risk factors from unhealthy eating behaviour which elevate blood pressure and serum cholesterol levels were reduced through a school-centered, multidisciplinary educational programme (Nicklas *et al.*, 1988). Social influences programmes in which students are taught social skills through modelling and rehearsal methods have been successful in preventing smoking in older children and adolescents (Botvin and McAlister, 1990).

Other studies have documented the ability of children with chronic health conditions to learn self-care. Lewis and Lewis (1990), for example, have demonstrated that children with asthma and epilepsy significantly improved their ability to manage their health problems through programmes which both increased their knowledge of their condition and involved them directly in their own health plan (Lewis and Lewis, 1990). Other progressive school health education programmes, such as the Know Your Body and Growing Health Curricula, are emphasising health promotion and are fostering the development of self-reliance and skill mastery in personal health habits (Lovato, 1990).

Empowerment: the barriers in the present system

The weight of the evidence cited makes a strong case for the power of a life-skills approach to health education as an effective and cost-efficient health promotion strategy. We know that children will adopt healthy lifestyle behaviours, at least temporarily, if we empower them through education. The questions to be answered now and in the future concern not so much the effectiveness of empowerment methods applied to children as individuals in improving their health, as they concern the very real difficulties of society's view of empowerment itself, and who is entitled to be empowered. Clearly, the permanent development of healthy lifestyle behaviours during childhood and adolescence, along with a personal valuing of being in charge of one's own health, is not only a complex but multidimensional process. Consequently, we must begin to examine the social and cultural expectations, and institutional factors that sometimes make the bridge between empowerment in theory and empowerment in actual practice a difficult one to cross. There are two primary obstacles to the empowerment of children in the field of health care. The first obstacle has to do with the developmental stages of children themselves. Children are not – and we sometimes need to remind ourselves of this in implementing health management programmes – merely small adults. What children are capable of understanding and the amount of responsibility for their own health they are capable of assuming at a given developmental stage are areas that need further investigation. The dangers of inflicting too much responsibility on children at a given stage of development, however, have been pointed out by David Elkind (1988) in an important book, *The Hurried Child: Growing Up Too Fast Too Soon*.

Elkind argues that traditional metaphors for the child, such as a child as the child as a blank slate or the child as a growing plant have been replaced today by a new metaphor, 'the superkid'. The superkid metaphor is particularly insidious because it inflates the stress already apparent in childhood, by creating demands for competence that children are not able developmentally to meet. Elkind says 'we are "miseducating" young children by teaching them the wrong things at the wrong time for no purpose' (ibid., xi). The superkid metaphor is significant for children's health issues because it illustrates the danger in overestimating children's competence at given developmental stages. Empowerment, as I have already suggested, is a valuable and necessary weapon in the fight for children's health, but it must be implemented developmentally, with due consideration of what children are actually capable of at a given stage. In order to understand more effectively the implications of empowerment for children at different ages, more research is called for. We need answers to questions such as the following:

- What are the specific health interests of children at different ages and what are their questions and worries related to these topics?
- How do children's questioning skills about health matters change over time?
- What techniques are most effective in determining a child's level of understanding about a particular health matter?
- Finally, what are the candid viewpoints of children and youth about lifestyle habits and more personal responsibility for their own health? In other words, how do children and youth interpret and rate the health lessons they presently receive?

My own experience with school-age children is that they often find health education materials boring, fearful, repetitive, too simplistic, moralistic in tone and confusing in terms of what the need to *know* and what they need to *do*. These are not the socially desirable responses we often get when doing formal programme evaluations. Nevertheless, girls and boys may be confirming Elkind's concern about the need for greater understanding of the developmental needs of youth when designing health education strategies.

The second obstacle to empowerment in children's health care, though related to the developmental issues just mentioned, is more systemic in nature and has to do with the conflicting messages that children take away from the health care environment. These conflicting messages arise from a fundamental problem within the model of empowerment itself. Hitherto, empowerment has been viewed primarily in terms of the individual. There is, of course, a certain amount of logic in viewing empowerment in terms of the individual because it is the individual's sense of control that impacts individual health. However, the individual always function within a larger social context, and it is the social context that frequently thwarts individual empowerment – especially with children.

In their research on health behaviours and the process of empowerment for children and youth in clinical settings, Lewis and Lewis were able to demonstrate that empowerment programmes do yield statistically significant knowledge gains and important behavioural changes, but that the diffusion of these interventions was impeded by several factors. In a recent description of their empowerment programme for children with epilepsy they noted, 'physicians were totally disinterested and unwilling to refer children with seizure disorders to a study designed to increase the competence of both children and parents'. In a follow-up to a health decision-making class, 'Actions for Health', the Lewises further noted that the attitudes of both parents and teachers interfered with children's abilities to gain decision-making skills.

Kamps *et al.* (1989) who studied parents whose teenage children had cancer, came to similar conclusions about parental attitudes to children's decision-making. The study concluded that parents were willing to let their children participate in the decision-making process related to the use of experimental chemotherapy; however, parents were more likely to overrule the adolescent if the adolescent decided against the treatment. This finding is consistent with the Lewises conclusion: 'Parents may be proud of their children and their accomplishments, but they are threatened by the competence of children and adolescents to assume an active role in the self-management of their chronic illness.' One assumes this uncertainty increases with more serious illnesses, but this is an assumption in need of testing.

Our own experiences with the HealthPact programme at the University of Colorado suggest that there may be many factors in the clinical situation itself that defeat children's empowerment. The HealthPact programme is a role development programme for health consumers of school age, designed to assist children and adolescents in developing certain social skills including a communication code (TLADD) for use during health care appointments. While working with the HealthPact programme, we attempted to gain insight into the feelings of third and fourth graders regarding their experiences in clinical health settings in Colorado and California. Seventy-five children were asked to draw a picture answering the question: 'What do you do in the doctor's office?' Children told their stories of waiting, being afraid and being left out in graphic detail. Most pictures had clocks. Many depicted passive, tiny, patient figures receiving gigantic shots from mean-looking doctors and nurses. Rarely did children draw themselves and health care providers talking to one another or jointly carrying out procedures.

It became obvious to us that genuine empowerment needs to go beyond the learning of social and communications skills. The very clinical environment needs to be made participatory rather than threatening. For example, receptions desks should be low enough that children can announce their own arrival. Health history forms must be adapted so that children as well as adolescents can be involved in the process of history-taking. Interactive health education material located in the waiting room should encourage active participation in the clinical experience. The significant interaction between doctors and nurses, or between clinicians and parents, which provide primary modelling experiences for children, must themselves be mutually interactive rather than examples of one person exerting power over another. In fact children have told me they have based their decision about the use of the HealthPact skills they have learned in the classroom on their observation of the type of dialogue that goes on between their own doctor, nurse and parents. That is when doctors and nurses, providers and parents do not have two way communication, the child is quick to realise the socially accepted behaviour for these settings is silence and cooperation. Even the books and toys children bring to their play to learn about the health care system reflect subtle but powerful messages. Children's books concentrate on explanations about what the health professional will do to you with little or no mention of the behaviour expected from the child. The implicit message is you have little if anything to do except cooperate. Doctors and nurses kits help children become oriented to what doctors and nurses do, but where is the consumer kit that orients boys and girls to their own role and responsibilities within and outside the health care system. The point here is not to eliminate the explanations about the health providers, but to balance it with stories and games that illustrate a more active role for the consumer beginning in childhood.

Encouraging empowerment

The intimidating and excluding language employed by health care professionals – in our case nursespeak – needs to be exchanged for a more mutually interactive style of communication that children can actually understand. Several studies have demonstrated that practitioners including nurses and children have difficulty communicating with one another; communication patterns of school nurses did not even acknowledge the child's point of view and provided children with only limited information. However, one investigation revealed that when asked, 92 per cent of the children studied revealed that they had a specific question directly relevant to the reason for their visit (Igoe, 1991).

Perhaps one of the reasons that the empowerment of children in health care has been approached through attempts to fix the child rather than the provider or the system, is that the child is easier to study, to educate, to affect than is the society as a whole. Even the modest changes in the clinical environment suggested above confront deep-seated social beliefs about the provider, child and parent relationships. However, if empowerment is to become a legitimate health promotion tool, the entire social–cultural context as it affects the balance of power for health issues must be confronted, beginning in childhood. The clinical environment and our position as health care professionals allow us to influence children's development of an active consumer role, as well as their commitment to healthier lifestyles, in unique ways. We have the authority of our professional position and we can either play this out in a way that fosters passivity or we can set the stage for developmentally appropriate self-sufficiency.

I suggest adopting a paradigm of empowerment for children's health issues similar to the one described by Wallerstein (1992) in a recent article for *The American Journal of Health Promotion*, where empowerment is defined not in individual but in group terms. She sees empowerment as an 'ecological construct that applies to interactive change on multiple levels: the individual, the organisation and the community'. Wallerstein continues by saying 'a study of empowerment, therefore, implies not just studying individual change, but also change in the social setting itself' (ibid., p. 198).

The implications for approaching individuals as a component of an ecological construct are subtle yet significant. Whereas the conservative view of empowerment focuses on the individual's acquisition of social skills rather than changing the conditions that create powerlessness, the ecological view takes all these into consideration. Proactive examples might include installing a suggestion box in waiting rooms of clinics and encouraging children as well as parents to participate in the improvement of these environments, or allowing students to help develop, organise and help teach their own lessons about healthy lifestyle habits.

Organisational empowerment, a term that derives from democratic management theory, emphasises the conditions within various organisations than engender the assumption of responsibility and decision-making by the individuals that make up the organisations. Organisations that empower their members can thus influence communities to promote system-level change. As individuals become proactive, organisations become proactive, and ultimately communities themselves become proactive. We, as nurses, as essential players in health delivery systems, have the power and the responsibility to initiate solutions from within these organisations as well as within our communities as citizens. According to Wallerstein (1992, p. 198):

> With this orientation, empowerment variously refers to communities achieving equality of resources; having both equity and the capacity to solve problems; identifying their own problems and solutions; increasing participation in community activities leading to improved neighborhoods, a stronger sense of community, and personal and political efficacy; and developing a participatory social action model to increase the effectiveness of natural helping systems and supporting proactive behaviors for social change.

The World Health Organisation (WHO) statement describing health promotion closely parallels Wallerstein's expanded definition of empowerment: 'a process of enabling individuals and communities to increase control over the determinants of health' (ibid.).

As an example of a proactive approach to empowering children in health care issues, the WHO has proposed the Healthy School Concept. A healthy school is defined as a community to which all children can relate and one that they have the right to change. The healthy school empowers children through its code of discipline, the prevailing standards of behaviour, and the interactive attitude adopted by staff with regards to students. An example of the healthy school approach adopted in Britain is a comprehensive health education programme called 'Health for Life' which spans both primary and secondary education. Empowered children have instituted many changes in their school including recycling programmes, a student-based system for conflict resolution, policies regarding smoking on campus and efforts aimed at drug and alcohol abuse (Kalnin *et al.*, 1992).

Through our own experience with HealthPact, a consumer health education programme, we have found that the social climates of families, schools and industries have a promising influence on the rate of adoption of PACT skills in the health delivery system. In a family, school or company which encourages participatory decision-making among students and employees, the application of a similar approach to a health setting becomes very effective once family members, students and employees have an understanding of how health systems operate and to what extent assertiveness produces results.

Organisational empowerment in terms of the health care system itself has been an evolving process. Initially, health care organisations were largely physician and administrator dominated. In the past two decades, however, we nurses have found our voice, and in many organisations have asserted our right to greater involvement in policy-making. Now it is time for consumers themselves to become empowered because of the situation that all too often defeats children in their efforts towards empowerment. We teach children in schools, in daycare and at summer camp how to increase their personal responsibility for their own health, yet too frequently the first message they receive in the health care system itself is to 'be quiet and cooperate'.

Ironically, one of the moments children are most teachable about health is probably when they are within the health care system itself – studies document the public's trust in the credibility of health professionals as health teachers. It follows then, that we in the nursing profession, who ourselves have direct experience in the difficult and sometimes painful struggle for empowerment within health organisations, are better positioned than most to assist consumers in their quest for control over their own lives?

An example of the proactive approach to children's health issues described here is the plan sponsored jointly by the American Nurses Association and the national league of Nursing Consumer Health Council. This agenda seeks to reform health care in the United States by empowering health care consumers of all ages to manage their own health matters with guidance from health professionals. But if agendas are to become realities, we must become even more active than we have been, within our organisations of course, but also within the larger community.

Promising programmes do exist, but for significant empowerment to occur, the individual, the family, the community and the health care delivery system itself must be made more responsive. More directed study as to how communities can be changed to enhance empowerment within health care systems is needed. But what is also needed, is for each of us, who have entered our profession out of a concern for common humanity, to be actively involved in the processes of change. You can make a difference in this regard and thereby assure healthier children for the twenty-first century.

References

ANA (1991). *Nursing's agenda for health care reform.* American Nurses Association: Kansas City.

Bloom, B. (1990). Vaccines for the Third World. *World Health*, June–July–August, 13–15.

Botvin, G. and McAlister, A. (1981). Cigarette smoking among children and adolescents: causes and prevention, in C. B. Arnold (ed.). *Annual Review of Disease Prevention*. Springer: New York.

Elkind, D. (1988). *The Hurried Child: Growing Up Too Fast Too Soon*, rev. edn. Addison-Wesley: Menlo Park, Cal.

Igoe, J. (1991). Empowerment of children and youth for consumer self-care. *American Journal of Health Promotion*, 6, 1, 55–65.

Igoe, J. and Giordano, B. (1992). *Expanding School Health Service to Serve Families in the 21st Century*. American Nurses Publishing, American Nurses Association: Kansas City.

Kalnin, I., McQueen, D., Backett, K., Curtice, L. and Currie, C. (1992). Children, empowerment and health promotion: some new directions in research and practice. *Health Promotion International*, 7, 1, 53–9.

Kamps, W. A., Humphrey, G. B. and Poppema, S. (Eds) (1989). *Hodgkins Disease in Children: Controversies and Current Practice*. Kluwer Academic: Boston.

Lewis, M. and Lewis, C. (1990). Consequences of empowering children to care for themselves. *Pediatrician*, 17, 63–76.

Lovato, C. (1990). *School Health in America: An Assessment of State Policies to Protect and Improve the Health of Students*, 5th edn. American School Health Association: Kent, Ohio.

Nakajima, H. and Grant, J. (1991). Universal child immunization: goal attained. *World Health Forum*, 12, 4, 493.

Nicklas, T., Johnson, C., Arbeit, M., Franklin, F. and Berenson, G. (1988). A dynamic family approach for the prevention of cardiovascular disease. *Journal of the American Dietetic Assocation* (November 1988), 88, 1438–40.

Shannon, B., Greene, G., Stallings, V., Achterberg, C., Berman, M., Gregoire, J., Marecic, M. and Shallcross, L. (1991). A dietary program for hyper-chlolesterolemic children and their parents. *Journal of the American Dietic Association*, 91, 208–12.

Wallerstein, N. (1992). Powerlessness, empowerment, and health: implication for health promotion programs. *American Journal of Health Promotion*, 6, 3, 193–205.

World Health Organisation (1991). *World Health Statistics Annual*, 23–7.

17 *Description of facilitative nursing interventions in primary health care: preliminary results*

Marjaana Pelkonen

Background and purpose of the study

In Finland the primary health care system based on the Primary Health Care Act from 1972 provides parents of under school-aged children with the opportunity of having regular contacts with public health nurses. This preventive and health promotive service is being used by almost 100 per cent of parents.

Various studies completed in the 1970s and especially in the 1980s indicate that interventions used in primary health care are not always based on the needs of the clients but rather on fairly standardised health education plans or old routines (Leskinen and Tossavainen, 1984; Kamppi *et al.*, 1988). In addition, there have been complaints that the functioning of public health nurses has been oriented too much towards the physical health of the child rather than the holistic health of the family. Background ideology has been identified to be somewhat authoritative rather than oriented to the concept of partnership. These factors hinder the development of good collaboration between clients and health care workers and do not promote health, for instance, encouraging initiative or self-control of the clients.

The mission of nursing includes the idea of promoting positive health (e.g. Smith, 1990; Meleis, 1991; WHO, 1991). Thus, it gives the impetus to foster the prerequirements of parents so that they can make their own decisions regarding the promotion of the health of their families. Prerequirements which include abilities and skills have been conceptualised as self-care resources in this study.

The purpose of the study was to compare the perceptions of families and public health nurses regarding the interventions public health nurses use to facilitate the development and use of self-care resources of the families. The ultimate goal is to develop facilitative interventions for the use of public health nurses in their practice, and also to extend the knowledge base about such interventions.

Background assumptions of the study are as follows:

1. Parents need various resources in order to maintain their own health and the health of their children.
2. The mission of nursing includes the enhancement of facilitation of the use of these resources.
3. To be able to enhance the resources it is necessary to employ a simplified approach and easy mediation which require the establishment of a good relationship between parents and public health nurses based on partnership.
4. In order to enhance the resources of parents, public health nurses require similar resources.

Conceptual framework

In the study, a framework based on the essential concepts of the child-rearing family resources and nursing strategy has been used. There are recognised similarities between this framework and Allen's model and ideology has been acknowledged (Krawitz and Frey, 1989). The family – as the focus of nursing – is defined as a unit of one or two parents and at least one child.

The self-care resources of the families were identified using Miller's (1983) concept of power resources. Power resources are characterised by the power inherent in every person and they gain expression through the ability to influence what happens to oneself. According to May (1972) the nature of power can be nutritive, manipulative, exploitive or competitive. The nutritive power used in this study includes the idea of caring about oneself and important others.

Power resources were modified and further conceptualised into six categories: physical health, social support, self-esteem, balance of energy, knowing and understanding, and belief system. These categories have been defined and given rationale according to the theoretical literature and relevant research studies. It has been recognised that the chosen way of conceptualisation is only one from many possible alternatives.

The facilitative nursing strategy includes three elements: a functioning relationship based on partnership between the nurse and the family; the interventions by which public health nurses identify, facilitate and help to develop the self-care resources of the families; and sufficient resources of the nurse which unable her to be effective. The interventions as well as the resources of the nurses have been grouped according to the above mentioned categories. However, a category of intervention aimed at building the relationship has been added.

Subjects and data

The subjects of the study were random samples of families of a 3-year-old child and public health nurses working with child-rearing families in health centres. The total population of families was approximately 60 000 from which a 4 per cent sample was drawn. The response rate of parents was 64 per cent (N = 1533). The population of public health nurses was 1400 and the sample size was 23 per cent. The final sample consisted of responses from 283 nurses, the response rate being 88 per cent.

Data were gathered by mailed questionnaires from both groups in 1991. Instruments were developed based on the three main concepts as a part of nursing strategy, and resources of the public health nurses. Thus, they included Likert scales for measuring resource and intervention variables, and questions for demographic variables. Intervention variables included perception of importance and experience of performance of each item. The intervention parts of the instruments of families and nurses were identical in order to make comparisons.

The instruments proved to be valid and reliable as measured by Cronbach's alphas. The alpha coefficients of the family instrument varied from .70 to .90. Corresponding figures of nurses were slightly lower. New combined variables were then computed for each category of interventions and resources. Resources were then grouped into three groups: sufficient, average and not-sufficient resources, and interventions into two groups: important–not important interventions, and performed well–not performed well interventions. The importance and performance of each intervention was then compared by using cross-tabulation. Explanatory statistics such as discriminant analysis have not yet been carried out.

Results

Description of the subjects

The majority of the families (95 per cent) had both parents and only 5 per cent were single-parent families, 90 per cent were official marriages and 10 per cent were open marriages. One-tenth of the families were step families. The numbers of children in each family varied between one and fourteen, with 50 per cent having two children and 20 per cent having one child and a further 20 per cent having three children. Education and social status of both parents were somewhat higher than in the Finnish population on average. The trend is clear: the younger the parents the better they are educated. However, all social groups were represented in the sample. Parents lived in all parts of the country, 60 per cent in cities and 40 per cent in the countryside which is in line with the distribution of population according to the census. Only 2 per cent were unemployed at that time compared to 5 per cent of the official statistics. The unemployment situation is now much worse. The majority of the nurses were married, had children and worked in all parts of the country, half in the cities and half in the countryside.

Sufficiency of resources

According to respondents, the resources of both parents and nurses were sufficient. The two best resources of the families were self-esteem and beliefs for the future and the two worst resources were energy and social support. The single parents felt that they had less support than the two-parent families. Respectively, the two best resources of the nurses were self-esteem and knowledge, and the two worst resources social support and beliefs for the future. The results also indicate that the good and bad aspects of life accumulate. The economic security was positively related to other resources. If economic security was not considered good, other resources were considered worse compared with those with better economic security.

Importance of interventions

In general, the interventions were considered important by families and nurses, although nurses valued all categories consistently higher than parents. Clearly, the most important category was building or maintaining a functioning relationship between parents and nurses. Next in importance were enhancing self-esteem and providing parents with knowledge so that parents could make their own decision. Least important was the idea of fostering the health of all family members in the child health clinic. However, both families and nurses indicated that the focus of nursing should be the whole family and not only the child as it mostly is today. Parents obviously want to be involved in the care of their children but they do not want interference in their personal matters by public health nurses. The majority of the families felt that they had hardly any opportunities to influence the services they receive.

Performance of interventions (considered important)

A general finding was that a clearly smaller proportion of parents thought that the interventions had been implemented well compared to the proportion considering the same intervention category important. Another consistent feature was that the public health nurses evaluated their performance to be better than the families did. Interventions considered to be performed best were building the relationship and enhancing self-esteem. Seventy-five per cent of parents considered enhancing self-esteem important and well performed and only 22 per cent though it was not performed well although it was important. Approximately 60 per cent of parents considered energy and social support as important, but they felt that the interventions by nurses to enhance them were poorly performed.

Discussion

Although the data analysis has not been quite completed, it can be said that the idea of personal resources and nurses fostering these resources is supported from these findings.

A positive result was that the relationship between parents and public health nurses was well established. In previous studies such relationships have been the focus of many complaints. Such a result gives a good basis for further developing nursing interventions in a more facilitative direction. The relationship is important especially because it is considered a major prerequirement for many other actions such as enhancing self-esteem.

The perceptions of parents and nurses regarding the importance of interventions were fairly similar which could be interpreted as an indication of similar values. It has been considered important to know the views of both clients and health care workers. Obviously, the potential for success is higher in these instances although constant validation of perceptions is needed in everyday nursing practice.

However, the major differences in the perceptions of parents and nurses were related to the performance of interventions. A question arises as to why public health nurses' perceptions were so much more positive than families' perceptions. Does this indicate a lack of sufficient evaluation or are parents more critical than the nurses?

On the basis of these results, it is clear that there is a major challenge to nurses. This involves developing interventions by which nurses can facilitate an optimal balance of energy and sufficient social support. This is not an easy task but on the basis of the literature there are many unused possibilities available for nurses to be deployed in their practice. Thus, the knowledge base of nurses needs to be reconsidered and further developed. It is evident that some nurses have adopted new ideas while others contrive to hold old values. This results in variations in quality which in turn can create an especially difficult situation when both the nurse and parents are provided with insufficient resources.

Further studies regarding resources are needed in which other categories and conceptualisations of resources can be employed. There is also a need to examine the relationship of interventions to outcomes. Focusing on the resources of parents and not on their behaviour allows parents to direct their own life and make their own decisions. Nursing could have a major impact in this development by being available when needed and working in a respectful and facilitative manner in partnership with families. In this way nurses will be contributing to the promotion of health and the principles of positive health.

References

Friedman, M.-L. (1989). The concept of family nursing. *Journal of Advanced Nursing, 14,* 211–16.

Kamppi, H., Makikarki, L. and Nummenmaa, M. (1988). Perheen tarpeiden huomioon ottaminen lastenneuvolassa, in Raatikainen, R. (ed.). *Hoitotyon tutkimuksia.* Kirjayhtyma: Helsinki.

Krawitz, M. and Frey, M. A. (1989). The Allen nursing model, in Fitzpatrick, J. J. and Whall, A. L. (eds). *Conceptual Models of Nursing: Analysis and Application,* 2nd edn. Appleton & Lange, Norwalk, Conn.: 313–29.

Leskinen, S. and Tossavainen, K. (1984). Leikki-ikasiten lasten vanhempien kokema hoito- ja kasvatusneuvonnan tarve seka lastenneuvolan, erityisesti terveydenhoitajan ossus perheen terveenhoidossa. Pro gradu-tutkielma. Kasvatustieteiden tiedekunta, Joensuun yliopisto.

May, R. (1972). *Power and Innocence: A Search for the Sources of Violence.* W. W. Norton: New York.

Meleis, A. I. (1991). *Theoretical Nursing: Development and Progress,* 2nd edn. J. B. Lippincott: Philadelphia.

Miller, J. F. (1983). *Coping with Chronic Illness: Overcoming Powerlessness.* F. A. Davis: Philadelphia.

Smith, M. C. (1990). Nursing's unique focus on health promotion. *Nursing Science Quarterly,* 105–6.

World Health Organisation (WHO) (1991). *Mission and Functions of the Nurse.* Nursing in Action Project. Health for All Series, no. 2. WHO Regional Office for Europe: Copenhagen.

18 *Towards healthier families*

Mary J. Renfrew

Introduction

The topic of health promotion for families is vast, covering, as it does, the health of mothers, fathers, children of all ages, and the extended family. This chapter will address maternal and child health specifically, although the principles that will be outlined may well apply also to other areas.

Women as key caregivers

The health of families in all countries revolves around the health of women, and their ability to care for other family members. Families, and the health of future generations, rely on women as the key caregivers in all cultures.

In most parts of the world, we are told by the Director General of the World Health Organisation, women plant and harvest most of the food, process and preserve it, carry the fuel and water needed to cook it, and cook and serve it. This is in addition to bearing, feeding, caring for, and clothing children, and nursing sick family members, both old and young. Women know that their own health and survival is essential for the health and survival of their families; children whose mothers die have a higher mortality rate than those who are cared for by their own mothers (Mahler, 1987).

The WHO Safe Motherhood Initiative has described how women and children are especially vulnerable to war, natural disasters and social and economic policies which increase poverty. Throughout all these events, women have to continue caring for families, and bearing and feeding children. Yet in all these circumstances, the first and most vulnerable victims are women and children. The League of Red Cross and Red Crescent Societies (1991) tells us that 'Women and children, far from being spared from the devastating effects of disasters, usually make up 70 to 80 per cent of those needing assistance.'

Recent events in Bosnia have brought home to us the impact of war on the welfare of families, especially children and women. Being closer, Bosnia perhaps has an immediate effect on us that similar events in the Gulf, Mozambique or Somalia may not have. We have seen men who have been separated from their wives and children, and women who have been left with the problems not only of protecting their children and themselves from the conflict, and from the brutal violence directed specifically against women, but also of finding food and clothing, and of giving birth under extremely difficult conditions. Difficult as it may be to accept, discrimination against women and children is often accentuated under conditions of extreme stress. A United Nations High Commission for Refugees official, commenting on the situation of Afghan refugee women in Pakistan, reported that she saw, 'Kilometres of people in need waiting in the cold to be registered, with the women last in line, some with bare feet in the snow' (League of Red Cross and Red Crescent Societies, 1991).

A recently published World Health Organisation document reminds us that 'the health, nutrition and lifestyle of women and the quality of care during pregnancy and delivery establish a foundation of physical health and intellectual and social development for the next generation' (WHO, 1992). These needs form the basis of an urgent health promotion agenda if we are seriously to address the health of future generations, because women face many profound challenges in trying to maintain the health of their families.

Problems women face

Around the world, half a million women die each year from pregnancy-related causes, including haemorrhage, infection and eclampsia (Kwast, 1991). These women, most of whom live in poorer countries, do not die because they have incurable diseases. Women in richer countries experience these problems too, but they seldom die from them. This is because they are protected by better nutrition and education, and because they have access to effective health care facilities, including family planning services.

The problem of maternal mortality is only the tip of an iceberg, however. It is compounded by morbidity or ill health among women who survive childbearing. Hard as it is to estimate the scale of women's suffering after childbirth, there is some evidence that in poorer countries, for every maternal death, there are sixteen women who suffer very serious disabilities such as vesico-vaginal fistula and severe anaemia (Datta, 1980). Many times more than this will have some form of suffering, such as a painful perineum, chronic backache, or depression.

One of the factors contributing to maternal mortality and morbidity is discrimination against girls and women. A World Health Organisation report tells us that unequal access to health care and food, excessive work at times of rapid growth, denial of equal opportunity for education, and obstacles to reproductive health, all leave a woman physically, socially and mentally unfit to exercise her full rights for personal and social development; and unable to protect herself from unwanted pregnancies or sexually transmitted diseases (WHO, 1992).

We need no evidence to remind us that women and young girls are subjected to discrimination in the richer countries, too, ranging from violence to a relative lack of financial security. Poverty is not confined to the poorer countries; a pregnant teenager in Birmingham, New York, Belfast or Sydney is likely to suffer problems of deprivation, social isolation and lack of potential for her future, just as her counterpart in Bangladesh is. We have seen some recognition of this with the recent UK Government target to reduce the incidence of teenage pregnancy (Department of Health, 1992a), although the need for special help for teenagers was not backed by support for increased benefits in a later government document (Department of Health, 1992b).

Primary care for families

Primary caregivers in the health services can do little to address such large-scale issues as widespread poverty, war and natural disaster. But primary care can offer a great deal to families, in the detection, prevention, and alleviation of suffering after childbirth. In the UK and other richer countries, maternal mortality rates are now minimal compared to those in poorer countries. We are faced, however, with the problem of widespread maternal morbidity. The limited evidence available suggests that the scale of this ill health is substantial.

A survey of women who had given birth in Birmingham, reported recently by Christine MacArthur and her colleagues (MacArthur *et al.*, 1991), is one of the few studies to assess the nature and frequency of chronic problems developing after childbirth. This large epidemiological study examined the postnatal health of 11 701 women in Birmingham, who gave birth between 1978 and 1985. Information was gathered using a postal questionnaire sent out in 1987 to the women themselves, and from their medical records. This study found problems to be very common. For example, a fifth of the women reported urinary incontinence at three months after birth. Ten per cent of women reported backache at three months, and this was nearly twice as common (19 per cent) among women who had had an epidural anaesthetic.

From this and other studies (for example, Sleep *et al.*, 1984), we have compiled a list of the most common problems women encounter after childbirth. These include perineal infections, perineal pain, dyspareunia, urinary problems, infections following caesarean section, breast infections, breastfeeding problems, depression, backache, headache, and bleeding problems.

Every year in the UK alone, hundreds of thousands of women who have given birth experience physical and psychological problems, many of which are chronic. A preliminary report of a large, ongoing study of women in the Grampian region of Scotland, six weeks after birth, concluded that 'the popular model of a healthy fit woman able to care for her baby is the exception. Most are tired, in pain, physically unwell, depressed or unable to cope well' (Glazener *et al.*, 1992). These problems must make the difficult and demanding task of caring for a new baby and the rest of the family impossible to do with the patience that is needed and the joy that it deserves. They have obvious short- and long-term effects on the health of the whole family. An exhausted or unhappy woman, with perineal or breast pain, or urinary incontinence, will look to her family for support. Her partner, her children, and her wider circle of relatives and friends are very likely to be affected by her illness.

The extent of this problem is hidden even from women themselves. Jenny Popay's research (1992) illustrates women's extraordinary ability to cope and their tendency to play down problems, often resulting in what might be called the 'Yes, I'm fine thank you' syndrome. Maybe it is no wonder that health visitors, midwives and general practitioners do not really know the extent of women's suffering. Women too often assume that their suffering is only 'normal', and that they should not complain. A former colleague wrote to tell us about her childbirth problems:

> As you have heard, things have not gone altogether smoothly . . . They are still pumping me full of antibiotics after both a womb and bladder infection and various other little problems. It was very unfortunate to have to go back into hospital and have a D and C. They put me on intravenous antibiotics for a few days with the drip in my right arm, and so I developed the art of folding and putting on a terry nappy with my left hand!!

Health workers, too, may risk the possibility of accepting serious problems as 'normal'. I recently reread an account of a woman's experience of trying, desperately,, to breastfeed her baby in the 1950s in London (Waller, 1946). 'A young woman told me that while struggling to give her baby the breast when her nipples were torn, she was rebuked [by a midwife] for letting her tears fall on its face. "But I was not crying at all, she asserted, it was sweat dripping off my forehead".' The author of this description, the obstetrician Harold

Waller, commented how women will often persevere in spite of intense pain and anxiety, in the interest of their children.

Our understanding of the problems that women face after childbirth has improved in recent years, but I am sure we can all recall times where women's problems have not been addressed with the kindness and understanding that they needed. Sore perineums after birth, sore breasts and nipples while breastfeeding, unhappiness after childbirth, are seen so commonly by caregivers that they may indeed come to be seen as normal. But they can present major problems for women and their families, with the potential for disrupting the early days and weeks after birth, when the family should be learning about each other, enjoying the new baby, and adjusting life to accommodate to the huge changes associated with the arrival of the new family member.

Part of the problem for caregivers is that we often do not know how to deal effectively with the problems experienced by women. What should we do for a woman with a very painful perineum, or severe breast pain? Where is the research that we need to guide us? There is a serious lack of research on the basic and widespread problems facing women after birth. In part, this reflects the assumption that these problems are 'normal', resulting in a lack of motivation to find out how to prevent or alleviate women's problems. And sometimes when caregivers do try to help after the damage has been done, for example by suggesting stopping breastfeeding when the woman has sore nipples, or taking the baby away to the nursery so she can rest, they can seriously compound the problem by undermining the woman's confidence and reducing the vital contact between herself and her baby.

Sometimes research evidence that is available to guide us is not used in practice. Holden's (1980) study of responsive counselling by health visitors for women with postpartum depression showed that eight weekly counselling visits greatly reduced the incidence of depression. In how many places is this service available to women who suffer from postpartum depression? Mental illness is stated to be a priority area in the 'Health of the Nation' White Paper (Department of Health, 1992a), and depression is one of the most prevalent forms of mental illness. I hope that the widespread unhappiness and depression experienced by women trying to care for their new babies and their families will now begin to receive the attention it deserves.

Women and their families need well-founded, available and appropriate support from the health services. These services must be flexible and geared to what families really need, not what we think they ought to need.

Breastfeeding and the family

To illustrate the general principles I have outlined, I want to consider the common ill health that women experience associated with breastfeeding. The scale of the problems women experience in Great Britain has been documented since 1975 in the five-yearly, national surveys carried out by OPCS (Martin, 1978; Martin and Monk, 1982; Martin and White, 1988). The Joint Breastfeeding Initiative was established in response to the levelling off of rates shown in the 1985 survey, and the importance of breastfeeding was emphasised in the 'Health of the Nation' White Paper; although it is notable that the emphasis was originally much greater in their Green Paper (1991). The government is setting up a national working group to identify and take forward action to increase the proportion of infants breastfed at birth and at six weeks. I am delighted to welcome this development. Nevertheless, the working group must look carefully at the real problems facing families and the caregivers who try to support women who wish to breastfeed.

It is widely acknowledged throughout the world that breastfeeding promotes infant health more than any alternative way of feeding a baby, regardless of country, culture or social background. It also has marked benefits for the mother, but only if it goes well. A recent World Health Organisation report describes in detail the nutritional, anti-infective, anti-atopic and contraceptive effects that result from women breastfeeding their own babies successfully (Akre, 1990), and an astonishing range of previously undiscovered qualities of human milk are still emerging.

Breastfeeding is difficult

There are understandable reasons why some women may choose not to breastfeed their infants (see, for example, Martin and White, 1988). These include cultural background and expectations (McIntosh, 1985), a distaste for breastfeeding, and difficult previous experiences, either of their own or of a member of their family, or of friends. Of the women who do choose to start breastfeeding, many have difficult or unpleasant experiences which may cause them to discontinue it prematurely, or perhaps to struggle on with breastfeeding in spite of difficulties (Houston, 1983; Martin and White, 1988).

In Great Britain, the most recent national figures available at this time (September 1992) relate to the 1985 OPCS survey: we still await the results of the 1990 survey. The 1985 figures show that, of the 65 per cent of women who started to breastfeed, nearly 40 per cent had stopped by the time the child was six weeks old (Martin and White, 1988). We do not know how many of those who continued did so in spite of problems and persistent difficulty. Information published recently in letters in the *British Medical Journal* give no grounds for reassurance that things have improved since 1985; a survey conducted in Fife in 1990 (Williams, 1992) shows that less than one in two women were breastfeeding on the tenth day after birth, and there appears to be an even higher attrition rate among Asian Muslim mothers in Birmingham (Stevenson, 1992).

Women describe a wide range of painful and difficult problems encountered as they try to feed their babies, including sore and bleeding nipples, mastitis, painful engorgement, and an inconsolable baby (Houston, 1983; Martin and White, 1988). Breastfeeding is difficult. It is associated with more depression and more fatigue and more broken nights among the women who choose to do it (Alder and Cox, 1983; Alder, 1984).

The pain and distress many women experience can be illustrated from the results of one of our recent studies. We have completed the data collection for a large randomised, controlled trial of treatments for women who want to breastfeed, but whose chances of doing so successfully may be compromised by inverted or flat nipples. We have not yet analysed the quantitative data, but we have read the comments that individual women made about their experiences in trying to breastfeed. Some typical examples demonstrate how hard it is for some women who want to breastfeed their babies:

> I had difficulties fixing the baby correctly which then caused the nipples to crack due to bad positioning. I used nipple shields, but my nipples cracked again when I stopped using them. The excruciating pain and seeing my baby bring up mouthfuls of blood was enough to put me off.

> My nipples were so sore I used to dread the next feed.

> Having had a caesarean and not feeling too wonderful anyway, I found it all too painful and exhausting particularly with an older child to look after as well.

> I was very upset and depressed at not being able to breastfeed properly. Also I hated having my nipples pulled about by so many different people. Also being told repeatedly to relax became irritating.

> My postnatal recovery determined my ability to breastfeed . . . I required an episiotomy . . . I had a third degree tear, and was stitched . . . initially breastfeeding was successful until the epidural wore off. I was unable to sit comfortably – the registrar had

stitched through my anal sphincter – disaster set in and after 4 days I was told by hospital staff to stop attempting to breastfeed as I was clearly 'not cut out to breastfeed'. No pain relief or treatment was offered to easy my pain.

These problems are not confined to women who have inverted or flat nipples. This last quotation illustrates again what I found in a study in the early 1980s, in Edinburgh (Houston, 1983). Women who want to breastfeed often find that other aspects of their lives and health, such as a sore perineum, backache or emotional troubles in the family, all conspire to make breastfeeding even more difficult.

It is not surprising that women often choose not to breastfeed. All these difficulties demonstrate that in the UK, as in many other countries, women do not have the choice to breastfeed that they and their babies deserve. They have a choice between bottle feeding and attempting to breastfeed, and encountering a range of painful and distressing difficulties.

And yet breastfeeding can be a pain-free, uncomplicated, joyous experience for both mother and baby, and that joy can spread to the whole family as both mother and baby are calm, peaceful and well rested. As women in many of the poorer countries of the world demonstrate, almost all the main complications of breastfeeding can be either prevented, or alleviated, with the right care. For this, women need to have good support and advice, at least from the very first feed onwards, and for the first few weeks after birth, from caregivers who are knowledgeable about breastfeeding and who have confidence in its success. Part of the WHO/UNICEF 'Baby friendly hospitals' campaign is for this kind of support to be available right from the very first feed (*Midwives Chronicle*, 1991).

Why is breastfeeding still so difficult?

Why do we still have serious problems in dealing with the distressing and common ill health associated with starting to breastfeed?

I cannot address the many interrelated factors in great detail, but it is important to recognise that this is an area where attitudes to breasts and sexuality appear to be important. The culture in which we live greatly affects how possible it is to breastfeed. For example, it is not easy to breastfeed in public. As the Joint Breastfeeding Initiative (1990) survey showed, four out of ten people disapproved of women breastfeeding in public places, and half of them disapproved of women breastfeeding their babies in restaurants. Women often have to overcome what seems to be an implicit but strong bias in favour of bottle feeding.

Women also encounter skills and attitudes in their caregivers, which range from skilled and knowledgeable, to uninterested and ill informed. It is not surprising that many midwives, health visitors and general practitioners have not developed the clinical skills to help women to breastfeed. Many were trained during the bottle feeding years, with misinformation which was based on the behaviour of bottle fed babies, and with a dearth of clinical skills to pass on to mothers and to new students. It is only in recent years that these skills have been acknowledged to be valuable.

As Garcia and her colleagues have described, women often experience dramatically conflicting advice which may or may not be accurate, and they often have no way of disentangling fact from opinion (Garforth and Garcia, 1989). As a consequence, the health professionals with whom women come into contact are not always truly supportive of breastfeeding. In a recently published study (Beeken and Waterston, 1992), 60 per cent of mothers said they were separated from their babies on the first night after birth; and breastfed babies were frequently given water to drink. Surveys from the UK, USA and Canada have uncovered a range of knowledge and ambivalent attitudes to breastfeeding among health professionals (Renfrew, 1988; Renfrew and Field, 1988; Anderson and Geden, 1991). One of these surveys, which I carried out in an English NHS district in 1987, strongly suggested that these ambivalent attitudes were aided and abetted by clever advertising campaigns for artificial feeds.

There are other factors which may influence the development of these ambivalent attitudes. One interesting suggestion by Lewis and Bradley (1992) was that caregivers are susceptible to their own personal backgrounds. They suggested that many midwives and health visitors were themselves bottle fed, and that 'Feeding a baby differently from the way we were fed means making implicit or explicit judgements on our own mothers: so midwives and health visitors are uncomfortable about making the mother they have in their minds feel guilty or inferior.'

The contribution of poor quality research to ambivalent attitudes

Another factor contributing to ambivalent attitudes among health workers and the public is the lack of good quality research investigating the health effects of infant feeding in countries with access to ample supplies of artificial milk and clean water, and about the effects of interventions such as additional bottles or timing of feeds, on the success of breastfeeding. In spite of the volume of research generated in this field over decades, many of the results of research in richer countries are conflicting, and many health workers find it understand-ably hard to muster the evidence they need to convince either themselves or others that there are marked advantages of breastfeeding in these countries (Cunningham, 1990; Labbok, 1990; Auerbach *et al.*, 1991). It would be fair to summarise the research literature at this stage which would leave us with more questions than answers about the relative effects of breast and bottle feeding in richer countries, and the relative merits of many treatments and practices. These questions can easily undermine the confidence of caregivers and of policy-makers in making clear statements about the superiority of breastfeeding, resulting in the 'breast is best, but . . .' syndrome.

How does this confusion arise? In recent years, I have been involved in systematic reviews of controlled trials relevant to the promotion of breastfeeding. These reviews first appeared in 1989 in *Effective Care in Pregnancy and Childbirth* (Chalmers *et al.*, 1989), and *A Guide to Effective Care in Pregnancy and Childbirth* (Enkin *et al.*, 1989), and updated versions of the reviews have been published electronically since then in *The Oxford Database of Perinatal Trials* (Chalmers, 1992). In the course of this work, it became apparent that breastfeeding studies are often of very poor quality, suffering from a range of methodological problems. These problems interfere seriously with the ability to derive clear answers to questions about infant feeding.

One of the most important flaws identified in these studies is the inconsistency in the term, 'breastfeeding'. As mothers know, babies vary widely in their feeding patterns. Some babies will be fully breastfed after they leave hospital, but might have been given bottles of formula and water for the first few days. Others might be breastfed, but have a bottle or two a day after the first six weeks. Another might be bottle fed, despite the mother trying to breastfeed for two weeks before giving artificial milk.

The realities of what babies and their families do, however, is not often reflected in research. For example, Dugdale, examining weight gain and illness in infants in 1971, defined as 'breastfeeding' any baby receiving any human milk. A bottle fed baby was one who received no human milk. The bottle feeding category was appropriate, but the breastfeeding category clearly included babies who received artificial feeding in addition to breastmilk. Frank and colleagues, in 1982, studied breastfeeding and respiratory virus infections. They defined breastfed babies as those who breastfed for at least three months, including those who were supplemented. Bottle fed babies either received no human milk or were breastfed for three weeks, or less. Both groups were therefore confused; breastfed babies received artificial feeds, and bottle fed babies received breastmilk. Auriccio and colleagues, in 1983, studying coeliac disease in children, defined breastfed babies as those who were breastfed for more than thirty days, while bottle fed babies were those who were bottle fed from birth, or who were breastfed for less than thirty days. In a final example, Agras and colleagues studied the early development of adiposity in 1987. They did not define either breast or bottle feeding. None of these papers found any advantage to the babies of breastfeeding – it would perhaps have been surprising if they had.

It is possible to carry out more accurate and sensitive research, reflecting what the baby's diet really was. A good example is the study carried out by Howie and his colleagues in Dundee, published in 1990. These researchers clearly defined the infant feeding groups, which included fully breastfeeding women (those who breastfed for thirteen weeks or more, and did not introduce supplements before that time), partially breastfeeding women (those who breastfed for thirteen weeks or more, but introduced supplements before that time), early weaning mothers (those who started breastfeeding but discontinued before thirteen weeks), and bottle feeding women (those who bottle fed from birth).

The results showed a clearly significant increase in gastrointestinal infections in babies who were bottle fed, or who were weaned early (before thirteen weeks), and this effect persisted up to one year of age. These results run counter to the often expressed view than in well-nourished populations, with adequate supplies of clean water, breastfeeding does not confer significant protection. Rather, this study demonstrates that with well-designed research and accurate analyses, breastfeeding can be shown to prevent infection in a British population.

Conclusion

Addressing the problems that women encounter during and after childbirth offers important opportunities to promote the health of families. Coping with a new baby is difficult enough, even without having to cope with a painful perineum, painful breasts, chronic headache and backache, and depression. The difficulties facing women are multiple, ranging from social deprivation and malnutrition to systematic discrimination and lack of health care. These problems are compounded by flaws in existing research, and a lack of research that examines the real problems that women and their families face. At the very least we should make sure that health care personnel do more good than harm, and that our advice is based on reliable information, not opinion.

Recommendations arising from this chapter

In addressing the multifactorial problems of breastfeeding in particular, and of maternal and child health more generally, we need:

Research

- Rigorous reassessment of all existing evidence, including systematic reviews
- Careful planning to ensure high quality of new research
- Communication between researchers, caregivers, women and their families, in the use of research results and in the planning and execution of new studies.

Clinical practice

- Available support and accurate advice for women
- Education of caregivers so that they acquire the knowledge and skills to help them understand the needs of their clients, and to work confidently with women

References

Agras, W. B. (1987). Does a vigorous feeding style influence early development of adiposity? *Journal of Paediatrics, 110*, 799–804.

Akre, J. (1990). Infant feeding: the physiological basis. Supplement to volume 67. *Bulletin of the World Health Organisation.*

Alder, E. (1984). Postpartum changes in mood and sexuality, and some implications for care, in Houston, M. J. (ed.). *Maternal and Infant Health Care.* Churchill Livingstone: Edinburgh: 70–91.

Alder, E. M. and Cox, J. L. (1983). Breastfeeding and postnatal depression. *J. Psychosom. Res., 27*: 139–44.

Anderson, E. and Geden, E. (1991). Nurses' knowledge of breastfeeding. *J. Obstet. Gynecol. Neonatal. Nurs., 20*, 58–64.

Auerbach, K. G., Renfrew, M. J. and Minchin, M. (1991). Infant feeding comparisons: a hazard to infant health? *Journal of Human Lactation, 7*, 63–71.

Auriccio, S. (1983). Does breastfeeding protect against the development of clinical symptoms of coeliac disease in children? *J. Pediatr. Gastroenterol. Nutr., 2*, 428–33.

Beeken, S. and Waterston, T. (1992). Health service support of breastfeeding – are we practising what we preach? *British Medical Journal, 305*, 285–7.

Blaikeley, J., Clarke, S., MacKeith, R. and Ogden, K. (1953). Breastfeeding: factors affecting success. *J. Obstet. Gynecol of the British Empire, 60*, 657–69.

Chalmers, I. (1989). Oxford Database of Perinatal Trials, version 1.2, disk issue 8, August 1992. Oxford University Press: Oxford.

Chalmers, I., Enkin, M. and Keirse, M. J. N. C. (1989). *Effective Care in Pregnancy and Childbirth.* Oxford University Press: Oxford.

Cunningham, A. (1990). *Breastfeeding, Bottlefeeding and Illness: An Annotated Bibliography.* Lactation Resource Centre, Nursing Mothers' Association of Australia: Melbourne.

Datta, K. K., Sharma, R. S. and Razack, P. M. A. (1980). Morbidity patterns amongst rural pregnant women in Alwar, Rajastan – a cohort study. *Health and Population Perspective and Issues, 3,* 282–92.

Department of Health (1991). *The Health of the Nation: A Consultative Document for Health in England.* Cm 1523. HMSO: London.

Department of Health (1992a). *The Health of the Nation: A Strategy for Health in England.* Cm 1986. HMSO: London.

Department of Health (1992b). *Maternity Services. Government Response to the Second Report from the Health Committee, Session 1991–92.* Cm 2018. HMSO: London.

Dugdale, A. E. (1967). The effect of the type of feeding on weight gain and illness in infants. *British Journal of Nutrition, 26,* 423–32.

Enkin, M., Chalmers, I. and Keirse, M. J. C. N. (1989). *A Guide to Effective Care in Pregnancy and Childbirth.* Oxford University Press: Oxford.

Frank, D. S. (1987). Commercial discharge packs and breastfeeding counselling: effects on infant-feeding practices in a randomized controlled trial. *Pediatrics, 80,* 845–54.

Garforth, S. and Garcia, J. (1989). Breastfeeding policies in practice: 'no wonder they get confused'. *Midwifery, 5,* 75–83.

Glazener, C., Templeton, A. and Russell, I. (1992). *Postnatal care in Grampian.* Aberdeen Health Services Research Unit. Occasional Paper (9 January).

Hoffmann, J. B. (1953). A suggested treatment for inverted nipples. *Am. J. Obstet. Gynecol., 66,* 346–8.

Holden, J. M., Sagorsky, R. and Cox, J. L. (1989). Counselling in a general practice setting: controlled study of health visitor intervention in treatment of postnatal depression. *British Medical Journal, 298,* 223–6.

Houston, M. J. (1983). Home support for the breastfeeding mother, in Houston, M. J. *Maternal and Infant Health.* Recent Advances in Nursing series, 49–69. Churchill Livingstone: Edinburgh.

Howie, P., Forsyth, J., Ogston, S., Clark, A. and du Florey, C. L. (1990). Protective effect of breast feeding against infection. *British Medical Journal, 300,* 11–6.

Hytten, F. E. and Baird, D. (1958). The development of the nipple in pregnancy. *The Lancet, 1,* 1201–4.

Illingworth, R. S., Stone, D. G. H., Jowett, G. H. and Scott, J. F. (1952). Self-demand feeding in a maternity unit. *The Lancet, 1,* 683–7.

Joint Breastfeeding Initiative (1990). *Joint Breastfeeding Initiative National Survey of Attitudes to Breastfeeding.* Joint Breastfeeding Initiative, National Childbirth Trust: London.

Kwast, B. (1991). Maternal mortality – the magnitude and the causes. *Midwifery, 7,* 4–7.

Labbok, M. and Krasovec, K. (1990). Toward consistency in breastfeeding definitions. *Stud. Fam. Plann., 21,* 226–30.

League of Red Cross and Red Crescent Societies (1991). Field Studies. Paper no 2: Working with women in emergency relief and rehabilitation programmes. LRC & RCS.

Lewis, E. and Bradley, E. (1992). (letter). *British Medical Journal, 305,* 523.

Mahler, H. (1987). The safe motherhood initiative: a call to action. *The Lancet* (21 March), 668–70.

Martin, J. (1978). *Infant feeding 1975.* OPC HMSO: London.

Martin, J. and Monk, J. (1982). *Infant feeding 1980.* OPCS, HMSO: London.

Martin, J. and White, A. (1988). *Infant Feeding 1985.* HMSO: London.

MacArthur, C., Lewis, M. and Knox, E. G. (1991). *Health after Childbirth.* HMSO: London.

McCandlish, R. and Renfrew, M. J. (1990). Development of the multicentre randomised controlled trial of alternative treatments for inverted and non-protractile nipples in pregnancy: the MAIN trial. *Research and the Midwife Conference Proceedings*, Glasgow and London, 21–4.

McIntosh, J. (1985). Barriers to breastfeeding: choice of feeding method in a sample of working class primiparae. *Midwifery, 1*, 213–24.

Midwives Chronicle (1991). 'Baby friendly' hospitals – new WHO/UNICEF initiative to promote breastfeeding. *Midwives Chronicle, 104*, 298.

Otte, M. J. (1975). Correcting inverted nipples: an aid to breastfeeding. *Am. J. Nurs., 75*, 454–6.

Popay, J. (1992). 'My health is alright, but I'm just tired all the time': women's experience of ill health, in Roberts, H. (ed.). *Women's Health Matters*. Routledge: London.

Renfrew, M. J. (1988). Developing midwifery research: the role of the midwife researcher at the National Perinatal Epidemiology Unit. *Research and the Midwife Conference Proceedings*, Glasgow and London, 86–9.

Renfrew, M. J. and Field, P. A. (1988). Practices and policies in the initiation of breastfeeding. *J. Obstet. Gynecol. Neonatal. Nurs., 17*, 418–24.

Renfrew, M. J. (1989). Giving free formula samples to breastfeeding mothers. Overview 4172, in Chalmers, I. *The Oxford Database of Perinatal Trials*. Oxford University Press: Oxford.

Rooney, C. (1992). Antenatal care and maternal health – how effective is it? WHO: Geneva. WHO/MSM/92.4.

Sleep, J., Grant, A., Garcia, J., Elbourne, D., Spencer, J. and Chalmers, I. (1984). West Berkshire perineal management trial. *British Medical Journal, 289*, 587–90.

Stevenson, J. (1992). (letter) *British Medical Journal, 305*, 523.

Waller, H. (1946). The early failure of breastfeeding. *Arch. Dis. Child., 21*, 1–12.

Williams, S. P. (1992). Health Service support of breastfeeding (letter). *British Medical Journal, 305*, 522–3.

World Health Organisation Report of the Director General (1992). *Child Health and Development: Health of the Newborn*. Forty-fifth World Health Assembly, Agenda Item 31 WHA45.22 March, WHO: Geneva.

19 Evaluating the impact of training community psychiatric nurses to educate relatives about schizophrenia: implications for health promotion at the secondary level

Charles Brooker

Introduction

This chapter describes one aspect of a three-year research project, funded by the Department of Health, which was conducted in the Department of Nursing at the University of Manchester. As the title suggests the study emphasises the value of health promotion for those already diagnosed as suffering from serious mental illness. The nurse's intervention is therefore pitched at the secondary level of prevention.

The main study examined outcome, in families caring for a relative with schizophrenia at home, after Community Psychiatric Nurses (CPNs) have been trained to deliver psychosocial intervention (Lam, 1991; Brooker *et al.*, 1992). At the outset it is important to look first, albeit briefly, at the context of the study in relation to the development of CPN-ing itself. The nature of the experimental training programmes in psychosocial intervention will then be presented.

Numeric growth of CPNs

The large increase in the CPN workforce over the last ten years is remarkable and associated, of course, with a number of policy issues, such as: the philosophy of community care, the closure of large psychiatric hospitals, and an intuitive feel that CPNs are, somehow, doing 'a good job'.

Emphasis in role

It is not enough just to know that, in crude numeric terms, CPNs have been increasing. What is of much more interest is to try and obtain some feel for what it is that they actually do! Historically, this was a simple matter, CPNs provided after care for those with serious mental illness on their discharge from hospital. This explains the marked preoccupation in the early CPN research literature with the role CPNs played in preventing the relapse associated with schizophrenia (Scott *et al.*, 1977).

There were critics of this role. Sladden (1979) looked in some depth at a team of five CPNs in Scotland, who, on average, had thirty-eight clients with a diagnosis of schizophrenia on their caseloads and concluded that 'nurses were at a loss as to how to deal with problems encountered in the family' and dealt with this stress by retreating into roles that were 'task-orientated' such as drug administration.

However, during the period 1980–90, there was a marked change in the role of CPNs nationally. The dramatic increase in the workforce coupled with increasing calls for professionalisation all led to a move away from 'psychiatry' (and all that this entailed) to the seemingly greener pastures of primary health care (PHC). Thus, by the end of the 1980s it was remarked that CPNs seemed to be dealing with the minor psychiatric morbidity known to exist in primary health care at the expense of those with long-term intractable problems (Wooff *et al.*, 1988). Indeed, Wooff described the CPN care of schizophrenia as consisting of 'very short contact times, the administration of depot medication and referral for consultant opinion when symptoms worsened'. These assertions have been shown to hold water across the country by the publication of the 1990 national CPN survey (see *Figure 19.1* and *Table 19.1*).

If the work of CPNs with clients suffering from a serious mental illness has been on the decline, has there been a policy response? The short answer is 'yes', central government has responded and in a variety of different ways. First, by the publication, in 1989, of the Care Programme Planning Guidance which demands that those referred to the specialist psychiatric services with 'health needs' are, at a minimum, assigned a key-worker, usually at discharge (Department of Health, 1989). Second, through the recent guidance to GP fundholders which strongly implies that care programme planning must be in place before such GPs can buy CPNs for other clients who are 'less severely mentally ill' (Department of Health, 1992). Finally, through the national mental health research priorities flagged up in 1992 by the

Table 19.1 *Medical referrals to CPNs correlated with category of client*

	Psychiatrist referrals	GP referrals
Proportion previously admitted	0.42*	−0.42*
Proportion 'chronically mentally ill'	0.39*	−0.39*
Proportion with a diagnosis of schizophrenia	0.33*	−0.33*

* P < 0.001
Source: Community Psychiatric Nurses Association, 1990.

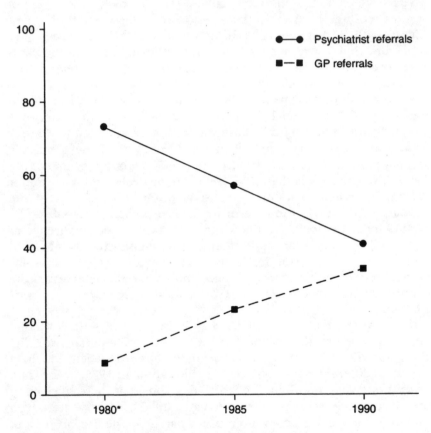

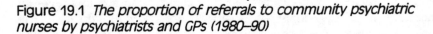

*Please note that the 1980 National CPN survey did not collect these data.
They have been extrapolated by the author from other sources.

Figure 19.1 *The proportion of referrals to community psychiatric nurses by psychiatrists and GPs (1980–90)*

Central Research and Development Committee (CRDC) which include the 'community care of the severely mentally ill'.

The nature of psychosocial intervention

So what is psychosocial intervention (PI)? Over the past decade the provision of social interventions to families caring for a relative with schizophrenia has been the focus of much research interest. A number of controlled studies have demonstrated that family intervention can reduce relapse and improve a family's quality of life (Faloon *et al.,* 1987; Leff *et al.,* 1989; Tarrier, 1988). Furthermore, it is clear that educating the family about the nature of schizophrenia is a core element of *all psychosocial intervention packages* (see *Table 19.2*).

In a major review of the educational methods used with families, Tarrier and Barrowclough (1986) demonstrate that a variety of educational techniques had been employed within the context of social intervention. First, the *simple deficit model* has been employed. This model assumes quite simply that a lack of knowledge leads to behaviour that is detrimental to health. The high levels of stress which can be found in some homes occur because relatives attribute the often bizarre and problematic symptoms of schizophrenia as somehow within the control of the client. *Ipso facto*, if these carers could be provided with information about the illness they would understand that this odd behaviour, far from being controllable, was often a likely consequence of schizophrenia. Thus, armed with this information, relatives could then modify their behaviour towards the sufferer.

On the other hand, the *interaction model* acknowledges the fundamental distinction between illness and disease by discriminating between the objective as opposed to the subjective. Disease is a paradigm of medicine and as such describes an *objective* pathology in

Table 19.2 *Component parts of psychosocial intervention*

- Detailed assessment of the family's life together
- Detailed assessment of each family members' needs
- Information about schizophrenia
- The design of a family-stress management programme
- Active encouragement to comply with neuroleptic drugs
- The creation of a 'working-alliance' with the family
- Psychological strategies for specific clinical problems

---

structure or function of the body and its associated organs (Eisenberg, 1977).

Illness, alternatively, focuses on each individual's *own personal and subjective experience* of disease and can therefore be influenced by a number of external variables, for example, personality, environment and cultural factors. As Helman (1981) has pointed out, people commonly use lay models of sickness both to comprehend and to cope with ill health in terms of their own circumstances. This model helps us to understand why, for instance, informal carers may hold a very strong view about the cause of schizophrenia.

Schizophrenia, in common with all forms of mental illness, is still heavily stigmatised and the behaviour associated with schizophrenia can be not only strange and often anti-social but also high in public profile. In other words, if your 18-year-old son is behaving in a very odd way that your neighbours cannot but fail to notice, you will, in the absence of a professional explanation, be driven to understand the cause. Unfortunately, this frequently occurs in a way that self-blames (see *Table 19.3*).

Implications of the interaction model of information-giving

The interaction model has important implications for both the content of family education programmes and the methods used to deliver such education as follows:

- If we adopt the interaction model the message to the family is that we believe information should not be given in a vacuum. Families need to be probed about their views concerning the aetiology of illness and the best ways in which to plan management. The client is the 'expert'.

Table 19.3 *Beliefs about the cause of schizophrenia*

- A man who believed that his son's schizophrenia began because he fed him melted chocolate

- Falling down and suffering minor head injuries, e.g. falls from bikes, downstairs, from trees, etc.

- Women often cite the fact that they went out to work was a major contributor and that the child care received was the cause

- Financial – not having the money to buy children the same as the other kids

---

- Families' views should be taken seriously but at the same time we should present alternative ideas that will improve the effectiveness of coping strategies, thus:
  - (a) Tailor information to the individual circumstance – do not focus on pathology in general
  - (b) Accept that views about illness may not change until other aspects of the intervention have been undertaken, thus PI (Psychological Intervention) is an important package of which information-giving is just one aspect
- Be selective about the information conveyed, use an understandable format and deliver it at a pace that allows absorption. Flesch reading tests have shown that some written information leaflets can only be understood by 12 per cent of the population!
- Actively and regularly evaluate the information that has been understood.
- Accept that the longer the family has coped with illness the harder it will be to effect change (and the lower the goals for change will be pitched).
- Give information in the most conducive environment with minimal distraction.

Thus, at a secondary level of prevention, the provision of information should be based on the interaction model which attempts to acknowledge: the tragic experience of families; their expertise (often developed in an *ad hoc* manner with very little systematic professional support); the crucial relationship between the reason for people's beliefs about illness and link between these views and their subsequent behaviour.

Method

A group of families who met standardised selection criteria were recruited to the pilot study (Brooker *et al.*, 1992). One group received psychosocial intervention from CPNs (the experimental group), the other, received standard CPN care (the control group). At one year follow-up, 71 per cent (n = 17) of the experimental families and 54 per cent (n = 13) were still engaged.

Data collection

The *functional value* of information possessed by a relative was obtained using the Knowledge About Schizophrenia Inventory or KASI (Barrowclough *et al.*, 1987). The KASI is a semi-structured interview guide which is rated by reliably trained scorers from audio tape recordings. The instrument assesses knowledge in the following areas: diagnosis, symptoms, aetiology, medication, prognosis and management. A global score of functional knowledge is also derived by summing scores from the six subscales. The KASI does not aim to assess *academic* knowledge about schizophrenia, but as explained above, examines the potential value of information in the management of the client's illness.

The subscales are rated from 1 to 4, where '1' indicates knowledge which may lead to detrimental behaviour on the part of the carer and '4' where the carer reports information which may lead to potentially valuable action in relation to the course of the client's illness, plus additional correct information.

The KASI has been shown to be quick to administer and good interrater reliability has been achieved. In the study reported here, the KASI was administered to the key relative in each family by both groups of CPNs at the following intervals: pre-intervention (baseline), post-intervention (six months after baseline) and at follow-up (a further six-month interval).

Results

The characteristics of the clients: The majority of clients were men (70 per cent) with a mean age of 33.1 years. Most were single (60 per cent), unemployed (90 per cent) and possessed no professionl qualifications (76 per cent). Two-thirds lived with either both parents or their mother alone. The formal psychiatric history of the group was as follows: mean number of psychiatric hospital admissions were 3.5; in total each client had spent a mean period of ninety-eight days in psychiatric hospitals. The average amount of time that had elapsed since the last such admission was 2.4 years and during this time all clients had been supported by a CPN for an average of 2.0 years. The diagnosis of schizophrenia had been confirmed by a psychiatrist prior to inclusion in the research.

The characteristics of the relatives: The average ages of the carers were as follows: mean age of mother was 57.5 years, mean age of father was 58.0 years, and (where appropriate) mean age of spouse was 36.8 years. There were no significant differences, between the groups at baseline, in relation to the carer's functional knowledge about schizophrenia.

KASI scores: At one year follow-up there were significant improvements in experimental relative's functional knowledge about schizophrenia in the following subscales: diagnosis, symptomatology, aetiology and medication (see *Table 19.4*). There were no changes in control group relatives scores. Similarly, the experimental relative's global score improved significantly whilst there was no change in the controls (see *Figure 19.2*).

Table 19.4 *KASI scores by group and measurement period*

KASI section	Median	Range	Z score	P value
Diagnosis				
Experimental – Pre	3	1–3		
Experimental – Post	3	2–4	–2.02	0.02*
Experimental – FU	3	3–3	–1.6	0.05*
Control – Pre	3	1–4		
Control – Post	3	1–3	–0.8	N.S.
Control – FU	3	2–3	0.0	N.S.
Symptomatology				
Experimental – Pre	3	1–3		
Experimental – Post	3	1–4	–1.15	N.S.
Experimental – FU	3	2–4	–1.96	0.02*
Control – Pre	2	1–4		
Control – Post	2.5	1–3	–0.33	N.S.
Control – FU	3.0	1–4	–0.73	N.S.
Aetiology				
Experimental – Pre	3	1–4		
Experimental – Post	2	2–4	–0.40	N.S.
Experimental – FU	3	2–4	–1.61	0.05*
Control – Pre	2	1–3		
Control – Post	2	1–3	–0.9	N.S.
Control – FU	2	1–4	0.0	N.S.
Medication				
Experimental – Pre	3	1–3		
Experimental – Post	3	1–4	–1.15	N.S.
Experimental – FU	4	3–4	–2.2	0.01**
Control – Pre	2.5	1–4		
Control – Post	4	1–4	–1.26	N.S.
Control – FU	3	2–4	–1.15	N.S.
Prognosis				
Experimental – Pre	2	1–4		
Experimental – Post	3	1–4	–2.11	0.02*
Experimental – FU	3	1–4	–1.42	N.S.
Control – Pre	2.5	1–3		
Control – Post	1	1–4	–0.36	N.S.
Control – FU	2.5	1–3	0.0	N.S.

Table 19.4 *Continued*

KASI section	Median	Range	Z score	P value
Management				
Experimental – Pre	3	1–3		
Experimental – Post	3	1–4	–0.63	N.S.
Experimental – FU	3	1–4	–1.18	N.S.
Control – Pre	2	1–3		
Control – Post	1.5	1–3	–0.84	N.S.
Control – FU	2	1–3	0.0	N.S.

Key
Pre   Pre intervention
Post After intervention
FU   One year follow up
*   Significant difference

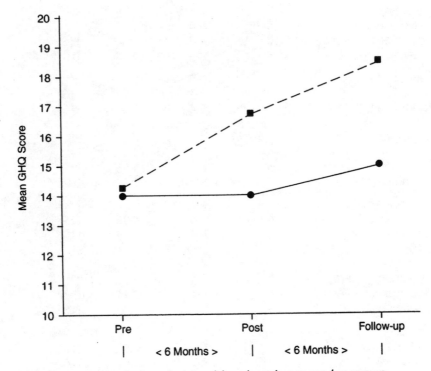

Figure 19.2 *Knowledge about schizophrenia scores by group*

Discussion

Educating relatives about the nature of schizophrenia is a crucial component of psychosocial intervention. It is a strategy that seeks to prevent further exacerbation of mental illness once it has been diagnosed. The purpose of providing information is to enable families to cope with the stress that is an undisputed feature of their home life by relieving them of some of their anxieties.

A number of educational approaches have been explored by researchers in this field including: individual family sessions; large group meetings with carers from different families; the use of video and booklets; even the distribution of information by mail. However, as Barrowclough (1987) and her colleagues have usefully pointed out such strategies are generally based on a 'deficit' model of education and therefore have shortcomings. Nurses, in their increasingly important role as health educators, may find the use of the 'interaction' model of information more effective. Certainly, the results reported in this study would suggest this could well be the case.

An 'interaction' model assumes that the acquisition of knowledge *per se* will not necessarily lead to positive changes in behaviour. The *emphasis must be on attempts to understand the reasons for people's beliefs about illness rather than focusing on pathology in general.* Ultimately, the information delivered will then be tailored to such individual nursing assessments.

The interaction model of information giving may have wider implications than the community nursing care of families caring for a relative with schizophrenia. In general, there is an ever increasing recognition of the relationship between stress and illness (e.g. in the community-based rehabilitation of coronary care patients), alongside a greater appreciation of the increased severity of illness with which informal carers are being expected to cope. The observation by Griffiths (1988) that the 'first task' of services is to support carers is clearly not yet borne out.

All community nurses, managers and educators might usefully consider the establishment of training/educational preparations which are underpinned by a psychosocial view of illness. Such courses could equip community nurses to provide families with information (based on an interaction model) and then to build on this first step by enabling families to manage the stress which is only too likely to occur at home as a consequence of chronic illness. Obvious though it may sound, illness does not affect just the client themselves but family and friends as well. A theoretical model which translates this recognition into the expert nursing care of families has been urgently required.

References

Barrowclough, C., Tarrier, N., Watts, S., Vaughn, C., Bamrah, J. and Freeman, H. (1987). Assessing the functional knowledge about schizophrenia: a preliminary report. *British Journal of Psychiatry, 151,* 1–8.

Brooker, C., Tarrier, N., Barrowclough, C., Butterworth, C. and Goldberg, D. (1992). The outcome of training community psychiatric nurses to deliver psychosocial intervention: report of a pilot study. *British Journal of Psychiatry, 160,* 836–44.

Department of Health (1980). The care programme approach for people with a mental illness referred to the specialist psychiatric services. HC(90)23/ LASSL/(90)11.

Department of Health (1992). *Extension of GP Fund-holding to Include Mental Health Services,* EL (92) 48. HMSO: London.

Eisenberg, L. (1977). Disease and illness: distinctions between professional and popular ideas of sickness. *Culture, Medicine and Psychiatry, 1,* 9–23.

Falloon, I., Boyd, J., McGill, C., Williamson, M., Razani, J., Moss, H., Gilderman, A. and Simpson, G. (1987). Family management in the prevention of morbidity in schizophrenia: clinical outcome of a two year longitudinal study. *Archives of General Psychiatry, 42,* 887–96.

Griffiths, R. (1988). *Community Care – an Agenda for Action.* HMSO: London.

Helman, C. (1981). Disease versus illness in general practice. *Journal of the Royal College of General Practitioners, 31,* 548–52.

Lam, D. (1992). Psychosocial family intervention in schizophrenia: a review of empirical studies. *Psychological Medicine, 21,* 423–41.

Leff, J., Berkowitz, R., Shavit, N., Strachan, A., Glass, I. and Vaughn, C. (1989). A trial of family therapy versus a relative's group for schizophrenia. *British Journal of Psychiatry, 154,* 58–66.

Scott, E., Shrma, S. and Temple, K. (1977). Care of the schizophrenic patient. *Nursing Times,* 19 May, 740–1.

Sladden, S. (1979). *Psychiatric nursing in the community: a study of a working situation.* Churchill Livingstone: Edinburgh.

Tarrier, N., and Barrowclough, C. (1986). Providing information to relatives about schizophrenia: some comments. *British Journal of Psychiatry, 149,* 458–63.

Tarrier, N., Barrowclough, C., Vaughn, C. *et al.* (1988). The community management of schizophrenia: a controlled trial of a behavioural intervention with families to reduce relapse. *British Journal of Psychiatry, 153,* 532–42.

White, E. (1990). *The Third Quinquennial Survey of Community Psychiatric Nursing Services.* Department of Nursing, University of Manchester: Manchester.

Wooff, K., Goldberg, D. and Fryers, T. (1988). The practice of community psychiatric nursing and mental health social work in Salford. *British Journal of Psychiatry, 152,* 783–92.

20 Meeting mental health education needs of patients: the potential role of the psychiatric nurse

Katharine Ferguson

Introduction

This chapter describes a small-scale in-depth study, exploring how a group of recently discharged psychiatric patients and their carers perceived their needs for education relating to the patients' problems and their care programme. The ability of nurses on the wards to anticipate these needs was also investigated, as well as their perceptions of their role in patient and family teaching.

The high relapse rate amongst people suffering mental health problems makes it vital that nurses are involved not only in 'patching people up' in times of illness, but that they are prepared to take on 'an advisory and supportive role to help people improve their quality of life and maintain their independence, whatever their state of illness or disability' (Kickbush, 1981). Whilst both patients and carers are recognised as having expertise by virtue of experience, there are likely to be gaps in their knowledge and experience. It is essential that these deficits are corrected as a basic right and to maximise their potential for self-care.

Literature review

Mental health promotion and education – a discussion

The fields of mental health promotion and education are very much in their infancy, being further developed in the USA, e.g. Caplan (1964), Ketterer *et al.*, (1980). A number of arguments can be lodged against the adoption of health promotion strategies in this field, most notably the failure, so far, to establish clearly causal agents of mental health problems, making preventive programmes difficult to focus. Causes, anyway, are likely to be multifactorial, so responsibility for prevention will fall between many different agencies. It is also argued that little can be done to alter the social factors which seem to be implicated in the aetiology of mental breakdown. The value of trying to 'teach' people to be mentally healthy may also be questioned. There can be no guarantee that education will lead to changes in behaviour.

However, a number of reasons can be cited for including education as a key part of the care programme for people in psychiatric hospitals, and their carers. These arguments can be divided into two broad categories:

- the 'person's rights' argument;
- the 'relapse prevention' argument.

The 'person's rights' argument

Both patients and carers have a right to full information on what is happening throughout the hospital admission, as well as needing comprehensive advice on the care programme on discharge, and how they can contribute to this. I think it is fair to say that patients' rights have often been neglected in psychiatric hospitals. Rosenthall *et al.* (1980) comment, 'Denial of information to patients amounts to what may be considered as denial of responsible adult status, and with it, the implication that the patient is not capable of intelligent choice and control.' With the move to community care, families are now providing the majority of care for the severely mentally ill. Goldman (1980) reports that 60 to 70 per cent of patients diagnosed as schizophrenic go home to their families after their first admission to hospital. Carers too have a right to information and advice.

The 'relapse prevention' argument

There is growing evidence that improving the quantity and quality of information and advice given to psychiatric patients and their carers may play a part in reducing relapse rates and improving quality of life. Caplan, in 1964, recognised education of patients and carers as an integral part of preventive psychiatry. Interventions, in this case, would be focused at the secondary and tertiary levels, i.e. teaching people to recognise symptoms and take action early, and helping the client achieve optimal function.

Research on compliance with psychotropic medication (a major problem amongst psychiatric patients, and a significant cause of relapse (Marston, 1970)), reveals the benefits of education programmes (Youssef, 1980). Pre-therapy orientation programmes have also been found by Larsen *et al.* (1983) to reduce drop-out from treatment. Work with the relatives of people suffering from schizophrenia strongly supports the value of education programmes in reducing relapse rates, increasing compliance and client satisfaction (Vaughn and Leff, 1981; Falloon *et al.*, 1982; Brooker, 1992).

Patient and family satisfaction with information and advice given in psychiatric hospitals

The research base on patient–carer satisfaction with psychiatric treatment is small. There is evidence to show, however, that patients frequently complain of not having received enough information on their condition and treatment, e.g. Ballinger (1971), Raphael (1977), Good Practices in Mental Health and Camden Consortium (1980), Sheilds *et al.* (1988). Most recently, the MIND report, 'People First', found 80 per cent of 500 people surveyed felt they had had insufficient information on their treatment. Carers, too, have reported dissatisfaction with information and guidance from hospital staff, particularly on how to cope with and best help their relative (Creer and Wing, 1974; Holden and Levine, 1982; Alstead, 1981).

The role of the psychiatric nurse in health education

Patient teaching is seen by many nurses and other staff as the primary responsibility of the nurse, e.g. Henderson (1966), Pender (1974), Caffarella (1984), Nelson *et al.* (1986). Butterworth (1991) states that education of patients and carers is an important area of development for mental health nurses, and should be an integral part of any nursing care plan. The 1982 pre-registration programme for mental health nurses made several references to the teaching role of the nurse, both in relation to patients and their families (National Boards for England and Wales, 1987). Project 2000 curricula, of course, also have a strong health education emphasis (UKCC, 1986).

In practice, however, there is evidence that patient teaching in hospitals is often still inadequate and occurring in a haphazard way. Cohen (1980), in a review of the literature, points out that although there appears to be a growing interest in patient education, including psychiatry, it is often an incidental part of care. There are very few studies evaluating patient teaching by nurses, specifically within the mental health field. Altschul's research in 1972, however, revealed that psychiatric nurses spent as little as 8 per cent of their time in one-to-one interaction with patients, and most of this was on an *ad hoc* basis. Cormack (1976) found similar results in his observation of the work of charge nurses. Communication with relatives averaged only 2 per cent of the nurse's day. Rarely initiated by staff, it tended to occur in public places and consisted in the main of 'superficial progress reports'. Miller (1983), in an Australian study, found psychiatric nurses tended to see patient teaching as their responsibility but were confused about which areas should be covered by nurses.

The study

The aims of the study were as follows:

1. To investigate the perceived needs for information and advice of a group of recently discharged psychiatric patients and their families, and how well they feel these were met during their last admission to hospital.
2. To investigate the ability of the ward nurses to anticipate their clients' needs for information and advice.
3. To explore nurses' views on their role as teachers of patients and carers.

Methodology

The samples were drawn from two acute psychiatric wards, and consisted of:

- All patients discharged from the ward over the four-month period of the study. Any patients identified by the nurses as being unfit to participate were excluded.
- The relative or friend most closely involved in the care of the patient.
- All registered nurses working day duty.

This was a 'convenience sample', in that it included all those subjects who were available over the four-month period, hence there are limitations in the extent to which the results can be generalised. Survey methods of data collection were used in the form of:

- Semi-structured interviews with patients, at home, within four weeks of discharge.
- Semi-structured interviews with the carers at home.
- Semi-structured questionnaires for the nurses, which were delivered personally by the researcher and collected from the ward.

Names of patients were collected weekly from the wards, and these were contacted by post requesting their participation. Following the interview, permission was sought from patients to contact their carers.

Results and discussion

Response rate

A total of forty-eight patients were contacted. A further nine either could not be traced or were readmitted, so were excluded from the study. In all twenty-three of the forty-eight agreed to be interviewed (47.9 per cent). The remainder were not at home or did not wish to take part. The low response rate is characteristic of follow-up surveys of psychiatric patients (Lebow, 1982; Munton, 1990), but may bias the results. A total of thirteen patients agreed for their carer to be contacted, and twelve of the families (92.3 per cent) agreed to be interviewed. The questionnaire was answered by eleven of the twelve eligible nurses (91.6 per cent response).

Perceived information and advice needs of patients

Patients expressed needs for advice and information in a range of areas, including diagnosis, prognosis and length of stay in hospital, practical advice, e.g. housing, finances, advice on how to cope out of hospital, medication and treatment, follow-up services, ward routine and orientation, legal advice, how to enjoy free time and relaxation. Individual patients differed in the specific needs they identified. No significant difference was found, however, between first and multiple contact patients, except that the former were more likely to need advice on coping after discharge. There was a close correlation between patient needs and those anticipated by nurses.

Perceived information and advice needs of carers

This group identified similar areas of need to those of the patients, with particular emphasis on how to look after their relative on a day to day basis and in times of crisis, and how to prevent relapse. Again there were differences apparent between individuals, although common themes emerged. Nurses were generally well able to anticipate carers' likely needs for information and advice, and similarly, specific needs were generally not met.

Patients perceptions of the quantity and quality of information and advice received in hospital

Whilst 30.4 per cent (n = 7) of the patients felt they were told everything they needed in hospital, 69.7 per cent felt that patient teaching was in some way inadequate. A total of 36.4 per cent of the patients (n = 8) were dissatisfied with what they were told about their hospital stay and 45.4 per cent (n = 10) with their preparation for discharge. In eleven out of fourteen cases, the fact that patients identified a particular need for teaching in an area, made them no more likely to receive it. On the one hand, 73.7 per cent of patients (n = 7) said they always or usually had to ask if they wanted to know anything. In contrast, 72.7 per cent of the nurses (n = 9) thought that patients always or usually got sufficient information or advice in hospital. Only 36.4 per cent (n = 4) of the nurses said they specifically set aside time for patient teaching, the majority tending to tell patients things 'as and when required'.

Family perceptions of the quantity and quality of information and advice received in hospital

Only one carer (8.3 per cent) felt they had been told everything they needed by hospital staff, comparing unfavourably with the patient sample (n = 7 or 36.4 per cent), and three of the carers (25 per cent) said they had had no information or advice at all. Surprisingly, though, satisfaction levels were quite high. Only three carers (25 per cent) were dissatisfied with information/advice relating to the hospital stay. A greater number, 58.3 per cent (n = 7), were unhappy with their preparation for the patient's discharge. As many as 91.7 per cent (n = 11) of the carers reported having to approach staff for information, and only three relatives had been seen privately.

A total of 66 per cent (n = 6) of the nurses (two missing), however, felt sufficient information was always/usually given to families. However, 72.2 per cent (n = 8) said they gave information/advice as and when required, rather than at specific times.

Sources of information and advice in hospital

Nurses were seen as the main source of information by both patients and families (*Table 20.1*). Nurses also saw themselves as having a major

Table 20.1 *Patients' and families' sources of information and advice*

Sources of information/ advice	Patients	Families
Nurses	20 (86.9%)	9 (75%)
Doctors	11 (39.1%)	4 (33%)

teaching role, either alone or alongside other members of the multidisciplinary team (the latter applied to most items). Although there was quite strong agreement that doctors should tell people their diagnosis and that nurses were responsible for ward orientation, there appeared to be confusion and disagreement about who was responsible for education in other areas.

Limitations

The nature and size of the sample, together with the low response rate, mean generalisation is not possible. It is also not possible to assess how much information clients *actually* received. It may be that the passage of time, exacerbated by effects of their illness and treatment, could have adversely affected patients' memories. Although nurses seem able to assess general needs for education, individual needs are often not met. Is this a failure to *assess* individuals or to *meet needs*? It is possible patients may have been afraid to criticise services for fear of repercussions (Jones *et al.*, 1987).

Recommendations for practice

The following recommendations are made:

1. Clients' (patients' and carers') needs for information and advice should be assessed on an individual basis, and a teaching plan drawn up, as part of the patient's plan of care.
2. There should be negotiation about how best these needs can be met, e.g. one to one, group settings, written information, videos.
3. The primary nurse should act as an information coordinator, both giving information and delegating to specialists. She also has responsibility for evaluating understanding and satisfaction.
4. Patient and family education should be more structured, with learning needs being reviewed at certain 'critical points', e.g. prior to leave/discharge, after ward rounds.

These recommendations have obvious resource implications, both in terms of necessary staff cover to improve communication practices, and the need for staff training in patient and family education.

References

Alstead, R. (1981). *Relatives of Psychiatric Patients – A Consideration of the Degree of Information and Support they Receive from Psychiatric Nurses.* Undergraduate research project. Kings College, London University: London.
Altschul, A. (1972). *Patient–Nurse Interaction.* Nursing Monograph, no. 3. Churchill Livingstone: Edinburgh.

Ballinger, B. R. (1971). The patient's view of psychiatric treatment. *Health Bulletin, XXXIX*, no. 4 (October).

Brooker, C. (1992). Training community psychiatric nurses for psychosocial intervention. *British Journal of Psychiatry, 160*, 836–44.

Butterworth, C. A. B. (1991). Generating research in mental nursing. *International Journal of Nursing Studies, 28*, 3, 237–46.

Caplan, G. (1964). *Principles of Preventive Psychiatry.* Tavistock Publications: London.

Caffarella, R. S. (1984). The nurse's role in a hospital based patient education programme for recovering adults. *Journal of Continuing Education in Nursing, 15*, 6, 222–3.

Cohen, S. (1980). Patient education: a review of the literature. *Journal of Advanced Nursing, 6*, 11–17.

Cormack, D. F. S. (1976). *Psychiatric Nursing Observed.* Royal College of Nursing: London.

Creer, C. and Wing, J. (1974). *Schizophrenia at Home.* National Schizophrenia Fellowship: London.

Falloon, I. R. H., Boyd, J. L., McGill, W., Rezani, J., Moss, H. and Gilderman, A. M. (1982). Family therapy with schizophrenics with a high risk of relapse. *New England Journal of Medicine, 306*, 1437–40.

Goldman, H. (1980). The post-hospital mental patient and family therapy: prospects and populations. *Journal of Marital and Family Therapy, 6*, 447–52.

Good Practices in Mental Health and Camden Consortium (1988). *Treated Well? A Code of Practice for Psychiatric Hospitals.* GMPH: 380–4 Harrow Rd, London W9 4HU.

Henderson, V. (1966). *The Nature of Nursing – A Definition and its Implications for Practice, Research and Education.* Macmillan Nursing: London.

Holden, D. F. and Levine, R. J. (1982). How families evaluate mental health professionals, resources and effect of illness. *Schizophrenia Bulletin, 8*, 626–33.

Jones, L., Lindermann, L. and Maclean, U. (1987). *Consumer Feedback for the NHS – A Literature Review.* King Edward Hospital Fund for London: London.

Ketterer, R. F., Bader, B. C. and Levy, M. R. (1980). Strategies and skills for promoting mental health in Price, R. H., Ketterer, R. F., Bader, B. L. and Monahon, J. (eds) *Prevention in Mental Health Vol. I.* Sage Publications: London.

Kickbush, I. (1981). Involvement in health – a social concept of health education. *International Journal of Health Education, 24*, 4, supplement.

Larsen, D. L., Nguyen, T. D., Green, R. S. and Attkisson, C. C. (1983). Enhancing the utilisation of outpatient mental health services. *Community Mental Health Journal, 19*, 305–20.

Lebow, J. (1982). Consumer satisfaction with mental health treatment. *Psychological Bulletin, 91*, 312–21.

Marston, M. V. (1970). Compliance with medical regimes – a review of the literature. *Nursing Research, 19*, 312–21.

Miller, G. (1983). Teaching psychiatric patients, in Wilson Barnett, J. (1983). *Patient Teaching.* Churchill Livingstone: Edinburgh.

MIND (1991). *People First.* MIND Publications: London.

Munton, R. (1990). What aspects of community psychiatric nursing does the client find satisfactory, in Brooker, C. (ed.) *Community Psychiatric Nursing: A Research Perspective.* Chapman & Hall: London.

National Boards for England and Wales (1987). *Syllabus of Training 1982. Professional Register Part 3. Registered Mental Nurse.* Bocardo Press: Oxford.

Nelson, D., Williams, S. and Villeneue, M. (1986). Assessing patients' teaching and learning needs. *Nursing Management, 17*, 5, May, 37–8.

Nutbeam, D. (1986). *Health Promotions Glossary: Health Promotion.* OUP 86, *1*, 1.

Pender, N. J. (1974). Patient identification with health information received during hospitalisation. *Nursing Research, 23*, 3, 262–7.

Raphael, W. (1977). *Psychiatric Hospitals Viewed by their Patients.* King Edward Hospital Fund for London: London.

Rosenthall, C., MacPherson, A. and Marshall, V. W. (1980). *Nurses, Patients and Families.* Croom Helm: London.

Sheilds, P. J., Morrison, B. A. and Hart, D. (1988). Consumer satisfaction on a psychiatric ward. *Journal of Advanced Nursing, 13*, 396–400.

United Kingdom Central Council for Nurses (1986). *Project 2000 – a Preparation for Practice.* UKCC: London.

Vaughn, C. E. and Leff, J. P. (1981). Patterns of emotional response in relatives of schizophrenic patients. *Schizophrenia Bulletin*, 43–5.

Youssef, F. A. (1980). Adherence to therapy in psychiatric patients – an empirical investigation. *International Journal of Nursing Studies, 21*, 1, 51–7.

SECTION FOUR

The nurse's role in promoting healthy lifestyles

It should now be clear that the philosophy of health promotion is fundamental to nursing. Providing resources, giving control and manipulating the environment positively are all part of this work. The related and more focused area of health education has already come under review in some chapters, so this next section demonstrates how the principles of health promotion can be integrated to improve the style and effectiveness of health education. Of primary importance to all health education is the realisation that there are almost infinite variations in the way that individuals respond to threats to health and illness and need to be supported. Without understanding an individual's feelings, perceived vulnerability, family support and motivation, information needs and range of coping strategies, interventions are likely to be insensitive and irrelevant. This is typified by McCaffrey's work with cancer patients and their recovery reflects this well.

In another area, cardiac rehabilitation programmes are amongst the most established, but they tend to be run in a way which reflects professionally organised sessions. Lessons on high-risk habits and perceived wisdom on what constitutes positive rehabilitation may be extremely helpful and certainly give opportunities for patients and significant others to have contact with those who may be able to help. However, fellow patients are often cited to be most helpful. This leads to the conclusion that it may well be the actual discussion of concerns and problems which aid adjustment and future independence. Certainly Foulkes' chapter seems to show this is the case for spouses.

Given that cigarette smoking, obesity and hypertension are the gravest risks for the affluent world, it is vital that research starts to explore the mechanisms by which preventive and rehabilitation or recovery interventions can be successful in moderating these. There is limited evidence that certain strategies based on discussion and advice are helpful to longer-term adjustment. More work is certainly needed to explore the process of such interactions. Rowe and Macleod Clark's study seems to suggest clearly that careful patient-focused communication can help to influence areas of behaviour change, such as cigarette smoking. Personal motivation and health belief seems to control patients' behaviour but the opportunity to explore these fully seems to be more important than a pre-planned educational programme which may reflect professional values rather than patient and family need.

Skills of communication and 'bringing out' the patients' and relatives' concerns are essential for this work. Growing evidence that nurse–patient interaction can be improved by more self-analysis of communication has important implications for continuing education. Each health carer should be able to understand the basic 'rules' of interaction and recognise their own deficiencies through tape recordings. This would not be expensive and given patients' or relatives' full consent both carers and future patients could benefit a great deal.

Underlying such skill is the belief that the patient or client should lead the way and become assertive in recognising needs and seeking support. Contrasts between some of the more traditional health education programmes and the progressive client-run groups, that use the health professional when they consider this useful, are impressive. Authors in the following section recognise that positive motivation and openness among participants is essential.

It is thus generally encouraging to note the change in principles underlying recovery 'programmes', these have now become more patient or family-focused and tend to advocate more control by participants. Where professionals are truly facilitative, their expertise is appreciated and probably can provide a positive element. Clearly health education is becoming less 'information' led and more sensitive to individual or group preferences.

21 Knowledge and distress: implications for cardiac recovery programmes

Joan Foulkes, Marie Johnston and Catherine Robertson

Introduction

Cardiac rehabilitation (CR) programmes aim to provide the patient and family with the information, skills and coping strategies necessary to take appropriate control over the management of their own recovery pain (Dorossiev, 1983; O'Connor, 1989; Thompson, 1990; Lewin *et al.*, 1992).

It is well recognised that a myocardial infarction (MI) can produce immediate and long-term effects which are physical and psychological in nature and affect both the patients and their families (Mayou, 1979; Wilson-Barnett, 1979; Cay, 1982). An MI is usually of sudden onset but stems from a chronic pathological state; this has implications in that the acute illness is often of a dramatic, but short lived duration. The patient and family may undergo a period of intense anxiety at the outset, at which time the emotional climate and problems of how people perceive their situation may influence their learning ability. Frequently, however, particularly since the use of thrombolytics, the patient's symptoms and physical condition may show a rapid improvement after initial therapy. It is then often more difficult for patients to believe that they have actually suffered a heart attack, indeed patients commonly say that they 'feel a fraud'. The short duration of symptoms and early discharge from hospital, sometimes after only five days, reinforces the belief that the episode was mild. Awareness and acknowledgement of the need for life-long behavioural change, in order to minimise the possibilities of reoccurrence, become less likely.

It is against this background that CR programmes have to work. As early as 1966, Henderson argued that it was part of the nurse's role to improve the patient's understanding and thus promote health. Cardiac rehabilitation addresses four major areas in the immediate post-MI period: (i) the patient's knowledge of the MI, the associated risk factors and recovery plan; (ii) their distress; (iii) the necessary modification of lifestyle; and (iv) the resumption of normal activities. The focus of this chapter is on knowledge and distress.

The results reported here are baseline data from the first fifty patients (thirty-two men and eighteen women) who entered a continuing study, the aim of which is to evaluate the benefits of structured educational CR programmes provided by a nurse counsellor for patients following a first MI (and their families). Patients were recruited within seventy-two hours of admission to the Coronary Care Unit at Ninewells Hospital, Dundee. Partners were also invited to participate. Ten patients were recruited on their own into the study as they did not wish anyone to be included with them. The mean age of patients was 57 years (range 41–70) and of partners was 53 years (range 28–71).

Knowledge

Knowledge has frequently been measured in order to evaluate the impact of patient teaching. Indeed some CR patient education studies appear to measure knowledge as an outcome in its own right (Rahe *et al.*, 1975; Owens *et al.*, 1978; Milazzo, 1980). However, a change of behaviour does not automatically result from increased knowledge of risk factors (Kemm, 1991) and knowledge should therefore be seen as a process, mediating a change in lifestyle, which is likely to reduce cardiac morbidity.

Even patients who are quite knowledgeable in some areas may have misconceptions which not only influence their post-MI behaviour, but may be a source of confusion and distress. A major component of the self-help Heart Manual designed by Lewin *et al.* (1992) was to provide cognitive approaches to assess and reduce misconceptions that were maladaptive.

The Knowledge questionnaire was constructed for the current study to elicit beliefs and misconceptions about a heart attack and resumption of normal activity. It consisted of nineteen items to which the response was True, False or Don't know. It was validated by an independent expert panel. Three separate scores were computed; a correct score, a misconception score and an uncertain score. The internal consistency of the scores was reasonable, the Cronbach alphas were 0.68, 0.57 and 0.74 respectively.

Several of the misconceptions which people reported may well have implications for their future recovery. Twelve per cent of the subjects in the current sample thought that the pain in a heart attack was known as heartburn, this incorrect belief may well result in either not reporting symptoms or causing them to try inappropriate analgesia. Sixty per cent thought that further pain always resulted in more actual damage to the heart; future anginal episodes may well cause greater distress for these people than those who made a correct assessment. Sixteen per cent believed that it was important to avoid laughing too hard after a heart attack! Other reported misconceptions which may impede resumption of normal activity included the belief that a heart attack means the heart is worn out, that after a heart attack most people never return to their previous level of activity and that sex life has to be modified forever.

Some misconceptions could result in an ill-advised recovery plan; 8 per cent thought that they should return to normal activity immediately on discharge, 9 per cent were uncertain about this. Four per cent thought that it was permissible to drive during the first week at home and 8 per cent were unsure. Fifteen per cent either disbelieved or were unsure that the chances of heart attack were less if they made necessary lifestyle changes.

No significant difference was found between patients and partners on either their total levels of knowledge or misconceptions. However, partners had significantly more uncertainty than patients.

Distress

Previous research suggested that both patients and partners would have high levels of distress (Mayou, 1979; Cay, 1982; Thompson *et al.*, 1982; Thompson *et al.*, 1987), and that women would have higher levels of anxiety (Vetter *et al.*, 1977). The psychological symptoms most commonly reported in the post-infarct period were anxiety and, to a lesser extent, depression.

The measure used for this study was the Hospital Anxiety and Depression (HAD) scale, a widely used questionnaire designed by Zigmond and Snaith in 1983 (cited 1990) to provide separate measures of anxiety and depression. It is brief and, unlike many other mood rating scales, items which reflect symptoms likely to be present in physical illness are, as far as possible, excluded. Scores of eleven or more on each subscale have been found to indicate the presence of clinical mood disorder.

Twelve per cent of the patients in the current sample scored above the cut-off point for clinical anxiety and only 2 per cent were above the cut-off score for clinical depression. By contrast, however, 60 per cent of the partners had anxiety scores above eleven and 20 per cent had depression scores above this level.

Patients in the present sample generally showed lower levels of anxiety and depression than might have been expected from the results of many previous studies (Mayou, 1979; Cay, 1982) where distress was assessed by psychological interview. The evaluation of findings in this area is confounded by methodological problems such as variations in methods of assessing anxiety and the different timing of the assessments.

Lower levels of distress have been found by several other authors, such as Sykes *et al.* (1989), who also argue that to focus on the means of a group may well be inappropriate as there are individuals within this whose levels are high. Havik and Maeland (1990) recommend that emotional reactions after infarction should be monitored during convalescence, as they have shown that for a subgroup of patients prolonged emotional upset may have a delayed onset. They argue that rather than follow the traditional concept of a linear relationship with emotional reactions resolving over time, they may actually follow a rather more complex pattern.

Having established that partners were more likely to be showing clinical levels of distress, it was plausible to ask if couples shared their distress. Did distress in one predict distress in the other? Results showed a significant correlation for anxiety but not for depression, i.e. couples tended to share their anxiety, but not their depression.

It was possible that partners were more distressed as a group because they were predominantly female (male = twelve, female = twenty-eight). Results, however, revealed no significant sex differences for either anxiety or depression. Male partners were as distressed as female partners and female patients had similar low levels to male patients. Vetter *et al.* (1977) demonstrated that female patients were more anxious than male patients, but this finding was not replicated in the current sample.

Association between cognitions and distress

In the nursing literature, several proposals about the relationship between cognitions and distress are discernible. First, greater knowledge, information or accurate expectations are expected to reduce distress. Second, greater uncertainty has been associated with greater distress. Third, some misconceptions, such as those addressed by Lewin (1992) may give rise to greater distress. These three hypotheses were examined in the current study. No association was found between total levels of knowledge, misconceptions or uncertainty and distress, although some individual items from the knowledge questionnaire showed some association with anxiety or depression.

Implications for cardiac rehabilitation programmes

The results from this early analysis have shown that partners, both male and female, are more likely to show higher levels of distress than do patients. Most of the previous research into partners of MI patients has investigated only the effects on wives (Cay, 1982; Hentinen, 1983; Thompson *et al.*, 1990), but the current research indicates that the high level of distress in partners affects husbands and wives equally. Families of MI patients often receive less attention from health care professionals, yet they play an important role in the patients' readjustment and recovery and in moderating the impact of the illness upon the family. These findings serve to emphasise earlier recommendations that partners should be included in cardiac recovery programmes. (Hentinen, 1983; Thompson, 1990). Spouses, family members and others having significant amounts of contact with the patient should be involved from the beginning because they experience their own difficulties in coping with the patient's condition (Wilson-Barnett, 1979), and because they may be particularly receptive to the need for their own lifestyle to change, with its potential for primary prevention, at the time of the MI (Hentinen, 1983; Thompson *et al.*, 1990).

The finding that patients had relatively low levels of distress may reflect the euphoria at survival, relief at being painfree or that patients were using avoidant coping, which whilst beneficial in the acute phase may lead to problems of adjustment if used in the long term. It is therefore important to measure changes in distress levels over the year following the MI and to assess ongoing coping strategies in order to monitor progress. This is being undertaken in the current study.

People in this sample have been shown to hold a varying range of beliefs and misconceptions which may have implications for future recovery. Ruzicki (1989) asserted that individual assessment is necessary as a guide to determining the educational needs of the person. The need for adequate assessment has been highlighted in several other studies (Casey *et al.*, 1984; Moynihan, 1984), and it has been shown that before meaningful patient education can take place one needs to know how the patient perceives the situation (Casey *et al.*, 1984).

As highlighted by Linn *et al.* (1984) there is now a move away from standardised information, dictated by the health professional towards an emphasis on the needs of the individual who may have diverse requirements. The results presented suggest that this information needs not only to be individually tailored for patients, but also to be adapted for the partners if maximum benefits of CR are to be achieved.

Acknowledgement

This research was supported by a grant from the Scottish Home and Health Department.

References

Casey, E., O'Connell, J. K. and Price, J. H. (1984). Perceptions of educational needs for patients after myocardial infarction. *Patient Education and Counselling*, 6, 2, 77–82.

Cay, E. L. (1982). Psychological problems in patients after myocardial infarction. *Advances in Cardiology*, 29, 108–12.

Dorossiev, D. (1983). Rehabilitation and comprehensive secondary prevention after acute myocardial infarction. Report on a study. *Europe Reports and Studies*, 84. WHO Regional Office for Europe: Copenhagen.

Havik, O. E. and Maeland, J. G. (1990). Patterns of emotional reactions after myocardial infarction. *Journal of Psychosomatic Research*, 34, 3, 271–85.

Henderson, V. (1966). *The nature of nursing: a definition and its implications for practice, research and education*. Macmillan: New York.

Hentinen, M. (1983). The need for instruction and support of wives of patients with myocardial infarction. *Journal of Advanced Nursing*, 8, 519–24.

Kemm, J. (1991). Health education and the problem of knowledge. *Health Promotion International*, 6, 4, 291–6.

Lewin, B., Robertson, I. H., Cay, E. L., Irving, J. B. and Campbell, M. (1992). A self-help post MI rehabilitation package – the heart manual: effects on psychological adjustment, hospitalization and GP consultation. *Lancet*, 339, 1036–40.

Linn, L. S., DiMatteo, D. R., Chang, B. L. and Cope, D. W. (1984). Consumer values and subsequent satisfaction ratings of physician behaviour. *Medical Care*, 22, 804–12.

Mayou, R. (1979). The course and determinants of reactions to myocardial infarction. *British Journal of Psychiatry*, 134, 588–94.

Milazzo, V., (1980). A study of the difference in health knowledge gained through formal and informal teaching. *Heart Lung*, 9, 1079–82.

Moynihan, M. (1984). Assessing the educational needs of post myocardial infarction patients. *Nursing Clinics of North America*, 19, 3, 441–7.

O'Connor, G. T. (1989). An overview of randomised trials of rehabilitation with exercise after myocardial infarction. *Circulation*, 80, 2, 234–44.

Owens, J., McCann, C. and Hutelmeyer, C. (1978). Cardiac rehabilitation: a patient education program. *Nursing Research*, 27, 148–50.

Rahe, R., Scalzi, C. and Shine, K. (1975). A teaching evaluation questionnaire for postmyocardial infarction patients. *Heart Lung*, 4, 759–66.

Ruzicki, D. (1989). Realistically meeting the educational needs of hospitalized acute and short-stay patients. *Nursing Clinics of North America*, 24, 629–36.

Steele, J., Ruzicki, D. (1987). An evaluation of the effectiveness of cardiac teaching during hospitalization. *Heart Lung*, 16, 306–11.

Sykes, D. H., Evans, A. E., McBoyle, D., McIlmoye, E. L. and Salathia, K. S. (1989). Discharge from a coronary care unit: psychological factors. *Journal of Psychosomatic Research*, 33, 4, 477–88.

Thompson, D. (1990). Counselling the coronary patient and partner. *Royal College of Nursing Research Series*. Scutari Press: London.

Thompson, D. R., Cordle, C. J. and Sutton, T. W. (1982). Anxiety in coronary patients. *International Rehabilitation Medicine*, 4, 161–64.

Thompson, D. R. and Meddis, R. (1990). Wives' responses to counselling early after myocardial infarction. *Journal of Psychosomatic Research, 34,* 3, 249–58.

Thompson, D. R., Webster, R. A., Cordle, C. J. and Sutton, T. W. (1987). Specific sources and pattern of anxiety in male patients with myocardial infarction. *British Journal of Medical Psychology, 60,* 343–8.

Vetter, N. J., Cay, E. L., Philip, A. E. and Strange, R. C. (1977). Anxiety on admission to a coronary care unit. *Journal of Psychosomatic Research, 21,* 38–73.

Wilson-Barnett, J. (1979). A review of research into the experience of patients suffering from coronary thrombosis. *International Journal of Nursing Studies, 16,* 183–93.

Zigmond, A. S. and Snaith, R. P. (1990). The hospital anxiety and depression scale. *Acta Psychiatr. Scand., 67,* 361–70.

22 *Evaluating the effectiveness of the coronary care nurses' role in smoking cessation*

Kathleen Rowe and Jill Macleod Clark

Background

In recent years there has been a growing awareness of the effects of cigarette smoking on health and in particular its correlation with coronary heart disease. It is estimated that smoking causes 110 000 premature deaths yearly (Doll and Peto, 1981). Coronary heart disease is the leading cause of death in the United Kingdom and in many developed countries, with Northern Ireland and Scotland having the highest death rate for this disease in the world. Approximately, one out of every four men under the age of 65 years die of coronary heart disease (OPCS, 1987). The effects of cigarette smoking on the circulatory system and in particular the correlation of smoking with the formation of atheroma in the coronary arteries has been well documented (Evans and Mathewson, 1986).

It has been emphasised that stopping smoking not only reduces the risk of coronary artery disease but improves the prognosis of those subjects who have experienced a myocardial infarction (Ball, 1972; Mulcahy *et al.*, 1975). Coronary mortality is halved in those who stop smoking following a myocardial infarction in comparison with those who continue (Ball, 1987).

This study was initiated in response to a growing concern of the needs of coronary care patients who may wish to stop smoking and the apparent gap in effective health education interventions in relation to nurses helping patients to change their smoking behaviour.

Macleod Clark *et al.* (1990), believing that nurses need a framework on which to base their health education interventions, adopted and modified a minimal intervention approach. The framework devised by Macleod Clark *et al.* was based partly on the Health Belief Model (Becker, 1974) and partly on the nursing process with which all nurses are now familiar (Kratz, 1979). It differs substantially from the minimal intervention approach suggested by Fowler (1983) in one respect, namely, that a heavy emphasis is placed on the assessment of each individual's knowledge and needs. Thus the intervention in terms of information giving and advice is tailored to the client's particular situation (Macleod Clark *et al.*, 1990).

This study was carried out to test the feasibility of using Macleod Clark's approach to individualised interventions to helping patients stop smoking in a coronary care unit.

Aims of the study

- To explore the smoking behaviour, health beliefs and degree of motivation to stop smoking of patients in a coronary care unit who had a myocardial infarction or severe attack of angina.
- To plan with the patient an individualised smoking cessation intervention including coping strategies and a support programme.
- To follow up patients in their own homes at three and six months and one year to assess smoking behaviour and allow experiences of stopping smoking to be discussed and further support to be planned if required.

The one-year data (*Table 22.1*) shows that seven (70 per cent) of the sample in the intervention group had ceased smoking. Two (20 per cent) had cut down by 40 and 50 per cent and one (10 per cent) dropped out of the study at three months.

Table 22.1 *Outcomes of intervention in terms of change in smoking behaviour at one year follow-up (n = 10)*

Sample	One year data intervention group Smoking behaviour
7 (70%)	Ceased smoking
2 (20%)	Cut down by 40% and 50%
1 (10%)	Dropped out of study

Method

Drawn from a population of clients within one coronary care unit in Northern Ireland, subjects in the intervention group comprised a self-selected, volunteer, convenience sample. All patients admitted to the coronary care unit during the course of data collection were invited to take part in an individualised smoking cessation programme. They were selected according to the following criteria:

- Diagnosis of myocardial infarction or severe angina attack.
- Under 65 years of age.
- Regular smokers who smoked at least ten cigarettes daily.
- Expressed a desire to give up smoking and agreed to take part in an individualised smoking cessation intervention.

Ten subjects (nine male and one female) meeting these criteria were allocated to the intervention group.

The nature of this study dictated that a case study design was most appropriate. However, it was considered valuable to collect some data from a reference group sample (n = 10). These were matched as far as possible to the profiles of the main study sample in terms of age, sex, social class, number of cigarettes smoked and length of time as a smoker, but they did not wish to receive the intervention. Within this sample, three were shown to have experienced a myocardial infarction and seven severe angina. They were advised to change their smoking behaviour and given a booklet on changing diet, stopping smoking, taking exercise, etc. (the standard procedure in this unit).

Subjects in this reference group were followed up at three and six months and one year at the cardiology review clinic. As all ten clients said they had not stopped smoking or changed their smoking behaviour, a verbal report of smoking behaviour was considered adequate.

The intervention

Interviews were conducted in the coronary care unit twenty-four to forty-eight hours after admission, depending on the physical status of the client. These were tape recorded in an attempt to minimise distortion bias through poor recall. A semi-structured approach incorporating open and closed questions was utilised. It encouraged in-depth knowledge to be gained in a natural setting and left scope for the researcher to 'probe' appropriate areas. It also facilitated the expression of feelings and attitudes through non-verbal cues and body language, allowing the researcher the opportunity of picking up areas of uncertainty not verbalised.

Smoking behaviour, health beliefs and degree of motivation to stop smoking were explored during the interview. A motivation check list was given to the subject prior to the taped interview. This indicated the desire to stop smoking and the determination and confidence to do so, and proved a useful guide to focus on problem areas. An individualised smoking cessation intervention was planned with the patient. After identification of needs, coping strategies were discussed, with the patient planning which strategy best suited his needs. It was vital that the patient explored the relationship between smoking and coronary heart disease and any potential problems with smoking cessation and also explored strategies for overcoming them.

A support programme was offered and all ten subjects requested a telephone link with the nurses. A nurse telephoned on a weekly or monthly basis as desired by the client and all subjects were aware they could telephone whenever they were experiencing a problem. All information about contacts was 'collated' by the nurses for the researcher. Carbon monoxide levels were recorded during the initial interview.

Subjects were followed up in their own homes at three and six months and one year by the researcher to monitor experiences of trying to change smoking behaviour, to offer support and encouragement and further advice if required. Carbon monoxide levels were collected at both three and six months and one year providing a source of encouragement to the subjects and some confirmation to the researcher of self-reported smoking behaviour. Carbon monoxide measures also acted as an educational exercise, in that subjects whose spouses or families smoked tended to have higher levels in their expired air from passive smoking effects. Salivary samples for cotinine levels were collected at six and twelve month follow-up visits to verify smoking behaviour objectively.

Data analysis

The interviews were transcribed by the researcher, and an analysis was undertaken based on what the subjects themselves said about their experiences and whether or not they found the intervention effective. Relationships were sought between patients' perceptions and behaviour change, and between the nursing input in the intervention and subsequent smoking outcomes.

Objective verification of smoking cessation was achieved by using a Bedfont Carbon Monoxide Monitor to record carbon monoxide levels in expired air, and by collecting salivary specimens for cotinine measurements.

Findings

To establish how effective the intervention was, the data obtained from the intervention group was scrutinised to see why some 70 per cent of the sample were successful in stopping smoking and some 20 per cent were not. *Table 22.2* shows the smoking behaviour prior to the intervention.

Table 22.2 *Smoking behaviour prior to intervention*

Category	No. of cigarettes per day	Mean	No. of smoking years	Mean years
Myocardial infarction 7 (70%)	35–80	49.2	25–40	31.4
Angina 3 (30%)	10–45	31.6	10–50	36.6

The data showed that the seven (70 per cent) of the sample who had experienced a myocardial infarction, smoked 35–80 cigarettes per day and had been smoking for 25–40 years, while the 3 (30 per cent) who had suffered angina smoked 10–45 cigarettes daily and had smoked for 10–50 years.

In so far as categorising the patients in relation to the number of cigarettes smoked and length of time a smoker, this factor was not found to be significant in this study. Light and heavy smokers were successful in changing smoking behaviour.

Motivation

The data were examined to discover if there was any difference in motivation between those who stopped smoking and those who didn't (*Tables 22.3* and *22.4*).

Table 22.3 *Motivation of patients who stopped smoking*

Patient	Responses to question: 'How much do you want to give up smoking?'
1	I definitely want to give up smoking, I definitely want to give up.
3	I do want to give up smoking.
4	I'd love to quit them altogether.
5	I want to give up smoking this time . . . I really do.
7	I-I-I'd just I-I-love to give up s-smoking.
9	Oh . . . I'd love to give them up.
10	I'd very much like to give them up.

Table 22.4 *Motivation of patients who did not stop smoking*

Patient no.	Responses to question: 'How much do you want to give up smoking?'
2	I do want to give them up but I'll do it my own way with a little help from you people if possible.
6	I want to give them up altogether.
8	I'd like to give them up . . . I would.

The findings show that those who gave up smoking were strongly motivated. While all three who did not succeed claimed to want to give up smoking, their motivation did not appear so strong. This expression of intent is significant in this study and indicates that no technique *per se* will help if the real problem is low motivation.

Internalisation

The beliefs of the clients and their acceptance of the link between smoking and coronary heart disease was examined. *Tables 22.5* and *22.6* show the degree of acceptance by both groups of the link between smoking and coronary heart disease.

The data showed that all seven (70 per cent) of the sample who stopped smoking accepted the link between their coronary heart disease. Whilst two (20 per cent) of those who did not stop smoking accepted that smoking affected their health, one (10 per cent) did not fully accept the link.

The fact that in this study there was total internalisation and acceptance by the seven subjects with myocardial infarction, to the belief that smoking did contribute to their coronary, must be recognised as an important cue to be utilised by nurses when planning post myocardial infarction rehabilitation.

Length of stay

Length of stay was compared between those in the intervention group who stopped smoking and those who did not (*Table 22.7*).

The data showed that the 7 myocardial infarction patients who stopped smoking stayed 7–9 days in hospital, while the 3 angina patients who cut down smoking stayed 2–3 days.

Length of stay was found to be a significant factor in that it provided the opportunity for maximum support and encouragement to be given in the initial stages of stopping smoking.

Table 22.5 *Internalisation of the link between smoking and coronary heart disease of those clients who stopped smoking*

Client no.	Responses to question: 'Why do you want to give up smoking?'
1	I got a real fright. The 'lights' were on the dim for me that Friday. They could have been switched out just as easy as that . . . Cigarettes did that.
3	It's essential for my health . . . I must stop smoking . . . I'll be dead if I don't.
4	This heart attack has made me want to give up smoking. Look what cigarettes have done . . . I slipped away you know.
5	Look what they've done to my heart.
7	Having this heart attack has brought it home to me, smoking does affect your health.
9	Definitely cigarettes have caused this . . . look, I even had a cigarette in my hand when it happened.
10	Well I've had a heart attack and if cigarettes can do that to me, I've got to take this chance now. I could have died that day.

Table 22.6 *Acceptance of link between smoking and coronary heart disease of those patients who did not stop smoking*

Patient no.	Responses to question: 'Why do you want to give up smoking?'
2	Well I say smoking does me 90% harm but 10% good, in that if I don't smoke at all it would affect my nerves so badly I might have a nervous break-down.
6	I have chest pain . . . the pain frightened me . . . it really hit me this time . . . it's the cigarettes . . . I'll have to give them up . . . I've got another chance.
8	They're no good for my chest . . . it's my breathing, I can't breathe.

Table 22.7 *Comparison of length of stay of those in intervention group*

Category of patients	Number of patients	Length of stay in days
Myocardial Infarction (stopped smoking)	7	7–9
Angina (cut down smoking)	3	2–3

Coping strategies

An important part of the intervention was the client's personal identification of coping strategies. These were utilised during times of temptation to smoke.

Tables 22.8 and *22.9* show a range of coping strategies identified by those who successfully ceased smoking and those who did not.

The data shows that all seven (70 per cent) of the sample who stopped smoking identified a range of both behavioural and cognitive coping strategies.

Whilst two of the three subjects who did not stop smoking identified coping strategies, one subject who dropped out of the study clearly did not.

From this study it was seen that identification of coping strategies played a significant role in the maintenance of smoking cessation. Both behavioural and cognitive coping mechanisms were utilised in hospital and following discharge.

Impact of the intervention

This study also identified that nurses' support had a significant impact on the smoking behaviours of the subjects. All subjects in the sample requested a telephone link or a visit. This link proved a vital support mechanism, both in maximising confidence levels and in talking through a crisis.

One subject experienced a life crisis following discharge. His brother died very suddenly, his wife and sons smoked and because he was so upset they offered him a cigarette. He said he was tempted and then he remembered the telephone link and rang the nurse and talked through his experience which helped and he did not smoke.

Table 22.8 *Self-support mechanisms as identified by those who stopped smoking*

Patient no.	Responses to question: 'What are you going to do if you are tempted to smoke?'
1	I'd do jigsaws to keep me from being bored. The main thing is I'll think of Friday 16th, the day I came in here – I think that will be enough to shock me into saying no.
3	If I can do without the first one in the morning, I think I'd be alright. Maybe something bitter in my mouth – a different taste – grapefruit juice.
4	I like walking but I would tell myself I've stopped smoking. I smoked my last cigarette on Christmas Eve. That's what I'd do.
5	I'd pop something in my mouth to take the desire away – a sweet – a sip of lemonade.
7	I'd nibble those small savory biscuits or have tea without sugar, then I'd be concentrating so hard in getting the tea down I wouldn't think of cigarettes.
9	If ever I'm tempted, I'll just think back to that pain in that store. That's the one thing I would think back to. I will never forget it.
10	All I need to do if I'm tempted is think about my illness. I don't want another Sunday like that again. My illness will be my biggest help.

Table 22.9 *Self-support mechanisms as identified by those who did not stop smoking*

Patient no.	Responses to question: 'What are you going to do if you are tempted to smoke?'
2	No there's nothing that would take a cigarette's place . . . sucking a sweet wouldn't help . . . something in your hand wouldn't help . . . I've no hobbies . . . I've no interests . . . I don't want any interests. I'll just figure it out somehow. I'll probably just cut them down.
6	I would try to get the desire out of my head. I would knit, or have a slice of fruit to take the desire away from my mouth.
8	I would go for a walk and count the money I'm saving up to buy myself a suit of clothes.

The impact of this study appeared very great in the identification and utilisation of coping strategies and in the nurses' support.

Comparison of data of the reference group with the intervention group

Data was examined to determine why seven (70 per cent) of the subjects in the intervention group ceased smoking, while ten (100 per cent) of the reference group did not change their smoking behaviour. The previous cardiac history of both groups was compared (*Table 22.10*).

The data showed that six (60 per cent) of the intervention group had no previous cardiac history whilst eight (80 per cent) of the reference group had. The intervention group had a total of seven previous cardiac admissions compared with forty-nine cardiac admissions in the reference group.

The findings in this study suggest that with repeated cardiac admissions, patients can become hardened to the warning signals. It is imperative to utilise an individualised smoking cessation intervention at an early stage in a client's cardiac history.

Motivation

Data was analysed to determine the degree of motivation of those in the intervention group who ceased smoking and those in the reference group who did not (*Table 22.11*).

The data demonstrates that 100 per cent of the intervention group wanted to give up smoking while only two (20 per cent) of the reference group said they would like to. All ten (100 per cent) of the intervention group were determined to give up compared with two (20 per cent) of the reference group who claimed they were fairly

Table 22.10 *Previous cardiac history of the reference group and the intervention group*

Previous cardiac history	Intervention group	Reference group
Yes	4 (40%)	8 (80%)
No	6 (60%)	2 (20%)
Previous cardiac admission	7	49

Table 22.11 *Motivation to give up smoking*

Intervention group			Reference group	
Desire				
I want to very much	8	80%	0	0%
I would like to	2	20%	2	20%
I don't know	0	0%	5	50%
I don't really want to	0	0%	3	30%
I don't want to at all	0	0%	0	0%
Totals	10	100%	10	100%
Determination				
I am very determined	7	70%	0	0%
I am fairly determined	3	30%	2	20%
Neither	0	0%	7	70%
I am fairly undetermined	0	0%	0	0%
I am not determined at all	0	0%	1	10%
Totals	10	100%	10	100%
Confidence				
I am very sure that if I tried I could give up	3	30%	0	0%
I am fairly sure	4	40%	0	0%
I don't know	3	30%	8	80%
I am fairly unsure	0	0%	1	10%
I am very unsure	0	0%	1	10%
Totals	10	100%	10	100%

determined. Seven (70 per cent) of the intervention group were confident they could stop smoking while eight (80 per cent) of the reference group did not know whether or not they could give up and two (20 per cent) felt they could not.

The findings show that the longer a person has a cardiac history and no smoking cessation intervention, the more resistant he is to change.

Cost effectiveness of the intervention

Cost effectiveness of the intervention was estimated in terms of cost per patient per day. It focused on readmissions during the six-month period following the intervention, and was estimated at £200 per patient per day (*Table 22.12*).

These findings support previous studies – Ball, 1972; Mulcahy,

Table 22.12 *Readmission in six months*

Reference (n = 10)		Intervention (n = 10)
12	1 Reinfarction 11 Angina	3 Angina

Cost estimated at £200 per patient per day

Length of stay		Angina	3 days
	—	Infarction	7 days
	—		
Total cost of readmissions	£8000 (Reference group)		£1800 (Intervention group)
Savings between reference group and intervention group			£6200

1975; Ball, 1987 — which suggest that post-myocardial patients who stop smoking have fewer admissions to hospital.

Discussion

In conclusion, this study assessed the feasibility and impact of using an individualised smoking cessation intervention in one coronary care unit. It found that patients who experience their first myocardial infarction appear more likely to accept the link between smoking behaviour and coronary heart disease than those with severe angina and long cardiac history. The combination of an acute coronary crisis and a stay in hospital provides an ideal opportunity to commence a smoking cessation intervention, but in the past this occasion has not usually been well utilised by nursing or medical staff. This study identified a group of long-term cardiac patients who, without individualised advice and support, had become a core of dissonant smokers — a practice which cannot remain unaddressed.

The individualised approach enabled the nurse and the patient to identify problem areas and consider appropriate coping strategies and support mechanisms, which were then employed following discharge from hospital. This approach was identified as highly appropriate for nurses working within a coronary care unit as a basis for their smoking cessation interventions. The impact of the intervention resulted in all seven post-myocardial infarction patients (70 per cent of the sample) maintaining smoking cessation at one year and two (20 per cent) of the angina patients cutting down the number of cigarettes smoked.

The intervention was found to be feasible in relation to nurse time spent, and highly cost effective because of the lower readmission rate of clients who had stopped smoking.

However, a deficit in nurses' confidence to carry out this important role of health education in relation to a smoking cessation intervention with patients was clearly identified. Nine of the ten interventions were carried out by the researcher, not from choice but due to a reluctance by nursing staff to carry out the interviews, as they felt ill equipped to do so. Interestingly, the one patient who was interviewed by a nurse maintained smoking cessation at one year.

Further research is now needed in order for generalisations to be applied beyond this case study sample. A training programme for nurses is recommended to enable all working within coronary care units to recognise their responsibility in assisting patients – especially first time myocardial infarction patients – to change their smoking behaviour. The study has identified a group of clients who, when first diagnosed as having a heart attack, relate the cause with their smoking behaviour and are motivated to stop smoking. The data suggest that the longer a person has a cardiac history with repeated admissions and no smoking cessation intervention, the more resistance is built against change. It is essential that nurses make effective use of their potential as health educators, in meeting the needs of post-myocardial infarction patients who smoke. It would appear that in this area those needs have been neglected in the past.

References

Ball, K.H. (1972). Cigarettes and the prevention of heart disease. *Rehabilitation*, 25, 17–20.

Ball, K. H. P. (1987). Stopping smoking cuts coronary mortality. *Health Trends*, 19, 11–13.

Becker, M. H. (1974). The health belief model and personal health behaviour. *Health Education Monographs*, 2, 324–508.

Doll, R. and Peto, R. (1981). *The Causes of Cancer*. Oxford University Press.

Evans, A. E. and Mathewson, Z. M. (1986). Risk factors in cardiovascular disease. *Science Progress*, 70, (4) 489–504.

Fowler, G. (1983). Advice against smoking: the attitudes of general practitioners. UICC Workshop on smoking cessation, Belfast. *Hansard*, 89, 30, cols. 138–9.

Janz, N. K. and Becker, M. H. (1984). The health belief model: a decade later. *Health Education Quarterly*, 11, (1), 1–47.

Kratz, C. (1979). *The Nursing Process*. Baillière Tindell: London.

Macleod Clark, J., Haverty, S. and Dendall, S. (1990). Helping people to stop smoking: a study of the nurse's role. *Journal of Advanced Nursing*, 15, 357–63.

Mulcahy, R., Hickey, N. and Graham, I. (1975). Factors influencing long term prognosis in male patients surviving a first coronary attack. *British Heart Journal*, 37, 158–9.

Office of Population, Censuses and Surveys (1987). *Socio Economic Group Based on Occupations*. HMSO: London.

23 Working with a women's slimming group: a case study of health promotion

Mary Malone and Liz Meerabeau

Introduction

This study of a slimming group formed in south-east London among the residents of a large local authority housing estate exemplifies differing perspectives on healthy eating and weight loss. Health educators have long concentrated on 'diet', that is on the food individuals eat, as opposed to 'dieting', which is a system of eating designed primarily to promote weight loss. Opinion varies as to the efficacy of advice on what constitutes a healthy diet; nevertheless, the belief that diet does indeed influence health remains potent among both health professionals and the general public. Charles and Kerr (1988) found that it is usually the woman rather than the man who 'stirs the cooking pot' in families with young children, although decisions on the content of meals may frequently be made by the man (Cline, 1990). Blaxter and Paterson (1982) have shown how beliefs about food and health can be passed from one generation to the next; thus, by addressing the issue of healthy eating within the slimming group, the health visitors involved could possibly hope to influence the dietary practices not just of the group members, but of their children.

Aims of the group

The group was formed in response to a request from local women, and followed on from a healthy eating campaign, initiated and led by local health visitors. In all, six group sessions took place over a period of three months. The health visitors aimed to use the slimming group as a means of addressing issues surrounding body image and self-esteem. Both were aware of the tendency towards what Shepherd (1992) calls 'fat fascism' within our society, and hoped that the slimming group

217

would provide support for women who felt vulnerable in relation to their own body image. Through discussion, it was hoped that group members would feel increasingly empowered to exert increasing control over their lives and, if they wished, over their body image. Depression and social isolation were also features of life for many women on the estate where the slimming group met, and it was hoped that these issues might also be addressed. The slimming group, then, was intended by the health visitors to have an impact on local women's physical, mental, psychological and social health.

The women who attended the group also had a very clear reason for doing so – to lose weight. Their attitude towards the health visitors' aims of increasing self-esteem and self-awareness is mirrored by Shepherd (1992): '*You* make peace with your body and I'll make peace with mine. Eventually. *When I'm thin.*' Weekly weighing became a feature of the group, and members wanted to count calories – nutritional values were mere optional extras. Success or failure was determined by the verdict given by the scales. On the insistence of the women, a weight chart was compiled. At one stage, a financial penalty for weight gain was requested which, given the stringent financial limitations of these women, showed how determined they were to lose weight.

The health visitors, however, saw such an unremitting concentration on losing weight as potentially harmful, and throughout the group's life a tension existed between the hopes and aims of the different members. Part of this chapter homes in on this tension; it aims to look at how health professionals may exploit the current fashion for female dieting and weight loss in order to meet quite different ends. This is not a new phenomenon, as Featherstone (1991) points out. In the late 1970s, the Health Education Council highlighted the cosmetic rewards of fitness and dietary care, as has the British Heart Foundation more recently. Thus, 'the body beautiful comes to be taken as a sign of prudence and prescience in health matters' (ibid., 183).

In spite of the tension which existed within the slimming group, one of the group's major achievements was to help the women involved become aware of certain external influences on how they felt about themselves, such as their partners, magazines, television and advertising. With this growing awareness came a determination to try to influence their lives and body shape *themselves*. This theme of empowerment also permeates this chapter.

Research method

The material for the study was gathered by the first author through a series of semi-structured interviews and by being a participant observer of the group process. Graham (1984) has shown how semi-structured interviews and 'story telling' can be a valuable means of collecting data from women. She describes how, for women in particular, there are aspects of our lives which 'cannot be shaped into answer sized pieces'. The issues involved were sensitive since, throughout the discussions, women were 'opening doors into their private lives' and could be potentially exploited. As the *narrators*, however, the women had at least some control over the story they told.

There were certain parallels between health visiting practice and the research process since the aim for both was to work in partnership, aided perhaps by the researcher's (then) status as a student health visitor. Other more personal attributes militated against partnership in 'fighting the flab', since the researcher was much smaller than most of the other women involved and resorted to a number of strategies such as wearing several layers of jumpers and flowing skirts on 'group days'. Certain forms of dress can, after all, 'declare the essential affinity between researcher and hosts without any attempt on the part of the former to ape the styles of the latter' (Hammersley and Atkinson, 1983, p. 79).

The researcher also went to some lengths to show that she felt under pressures similar to those which other group members experienced. As Cline (1990, p. 108) says about the whole ideology surrounding women, body image and food: 'understanding how a system (in this case the patriarchy which defines thin as beautiful) works does not necessarily prevent us being controlled by an ideological hold on our consciousness'.

The data suggest that the trust of the women within the group was perhaps won.

Literature review: women and food

There is a plethora of works, both scholarly and literary, concerning the rôle of food within a given society and the often problematic relationship women have with food. As Murcott (1983, p. 2) observes, 'Good food is more than a matter of nutritional value – a balanced diet is more than just a matter of health.'

Fieldhouse (1986) points to the cultural basis of food choice and the fact that foodstuffs considered edible in one culture are inedible in another. Moreover, it is not just what we choose to eat but *when and how* we eat it which is culturally prescribed (James, 1990). Foods which are 'good for you' are seen as less desirable whereas James asserts that 'bad' food has come to symbolise pleasure: hence the now rather dated advertisement for cream cakes which were 'naughty but nice'. For Coward (1984) luscious pictures of food may provide a clandestine pleasure for weight conscious women, in the same way that pornographic literature is said to do for some men.

Within the literary sphere, Margaret Atwood's first novel, *The Edible Woman*, tells the story of a young woman who becomes progressively unable to eat as her longed-for marriage approaches. The climax of the story involves the preparation of a cake, made in her own image, which is then eaten by one of her suitors. In *Life Size*, Jennifer Shute tells the story of a young, hospitalised anorexic woman, while Lucy Ellman in *Sweet Desserts* narrates the life stories of two women for whom life changes drastically over the years. All that remains constant is the comfort to be obtained from food.

Feminist writers such as Cline (1990), Orbach (1978) and Wolf (1990) have examined the political and psychological issues which they believe surround women, food and body image within our society. For Orbach, fat is a response to the inequality of the sexes, whereas Cline believes that food symbolises women's emotional needs and constitutes a language of both joy and anguish. Wolf (1990, p. 186) claims that dieting is a powerful 'political sedative' and that it counters 'the historical groundswell of female success with a mass conviction of female failure'.

Body image and the consumer culture

Featherstone (1982) describes the growth of the consumer culture in which the body should approximate to an idealised image of youth, health and beauty. This has been heightened by the advent of photography and particularly the video camera, so that we are now to some extent all performers, putting emphasis upon appearance, display and the management of impressions. Both Berger (1972) and Cline (1990) emphasise that women are particularly affected by this 'insidious controlling inspection' in which 'women watch themselves being looked at' (Berger, 1972).

For Featherstone (1982, p. 22) the body has come to be seen as a machine, as image which is, of course, currently being used in promoting 'The Health of the Nation'. Within our culture, he claims there is a tendency for 'ascribed body qualities to become regarded as plastic – with effort and body work individuals are persuaded they can achieve a certain desired appearance'.

The individual's appearance may thus come to be seen as a reflection of the inner self and its deficits an indication of laziness, low self-esteem or even moral failure. There is thus a danger that health educators, in promoting dietary changes and exercise regimes, may collude with the social dictate of 'the Look' and the notions of morality which surround it.

Research findings – body image

Most of the women felt very negative about their body shape. As one said: 'I felt awful. I've never been so *fat* before. I think people look at me, and they think how could she have let that happen.' Another said: 'If only I could lose a bit there [waist] and there [thighs], then I'd feel decent again. Like a proper woman, I'd be more confident too.'

Several women suggested that being fat both resulted in and reflected their lack of success in life:

> It's hard when you're fat. I used to go for jobs and I'd sit there thinking they won't give *me* this job. They'll give it to some dolly, some slim girl. It's nicer to look at her than at a big lump like me. Sure enough, I wouldn't get that job – not that I blame them really.

A further comment from this same woman about her friend's children indicated how closely body size and success were interlinked in her mind: 'They're really big and fat and they can't do a thing – big lumps! Look at her [daughter]. She's like a little rabbit. She's almost walking now and she's into everything.'

Guilt and lack of will power

Many women described their shame in relation to their eating and body shape:

> I'm on a diet now so that I'll be thin in the summer. I don't want to be ashamed when it's hot – all my bulges on display.

> It's no good blaming anyone else. It's my own fault I'm so big. I've got no control, have I? Well I'll start eating a bar of chocolate and I can't stop. I'll have to eat the whole thing. Piggery! I'm ashamed of myself.

For another woman,

> Being like this, being fat I mean, is a sign that I've let myself go. Got no self-control. You know how it is. I'll be in the house of an evening. He [husband] will have gone off for a drink and I'll think what's in the fridge. If it's a cake or something nice, I'll eat it all. It's for comfort really, I suppose.

Guilt was a theme which reverberated throughout all the interviews. Several women ate sweets and cakes only when there was no one else around; others were defensive about their secret pleasures. This suggests that many women, without any recognised eating disorder, obtain a guilty pleasure from food in secret.

Sexuality

Cline (1990) says that one of the myths about fatness is that fat women are not sexual beings. Several of the women in this study reflected this. One had recently married a man much younger than herself: 'I want to be thin and sexy. When you're like this, fat, you just don't feel that way. You feel like a blob'. Another said: 'When you're like this you're not like a woman. You're just fat. My husband says don't worry, but I *do*.'

The period after Christmas was a particularly difficult one for the slimming group. The mood was one of gloom and despondency, since the excesses of the festive season had now to be paid for by months of self-restraint. The word 'slob' was commonly used by women to describe themselves and some did not come to be weighed until they felt they had lost some of their extra pounds.

The final session

At this point it seemed as if the original health visiting aim of addressing issues surrounding women's physical, mental, emotional and social health was lost beneath the compulsion to become slim. Happily, this was not completely the case. The final group session did display something rather heartening, whereas the previous five sessions had concentrated on weight loss or gain, feelings of low self-esteem, guilt, and at times shame and self-disgust.

Perhaps, significantly, the final meeting took place in the community centre. There were no scales to be seen, so no one could be weighed. This time the group was joined by a very slim woman sipping black coffee who said she wanted to be a size 10. Another woman retorted that she was already like a rake, but, 'I know it's not your fault, love. They all tell you that you should lose weight. Even thin girls like you believe it.' When asked who 'they' were, she replied, 'You know, the telly, the papers, the adverts – everyone really. Nothing but pressure on you to look thin.'

This opened the floodgates for other group members to express their feelings:

You can't pick up a paper without some new faddy diet.

You don't see fat women on the telly. Only comedians. They must think it's funny to be fat.

I don't know who he [husband] thinks he is, telling me to lose weight, him with that beer belly.

He wants me to be thin but he also wants me to go for a few drinks with him and then for a curry afterwards. That puts paid to my diet. I can't win.

Let's face it. We're our own worst enemies, counting calories and looking at each other to see who's lost most weight.

This brief episode constituted the first glimmer of a new awareness of the pressures on women to adhere to a certain (thin) female form. The comments were quite different from those earlier expressions of guilt, of fear and of being trapped in their relationships with food. One woman even identified an element of rebellion: 'Sometimes I think I'm fat because I'm sick and tired of being told to be thin.'

With the now expressed hint of self-awareness among group members came the possibility of a growing determination to try to influence their lives and body shape *themselves*. This would surely be the first step on the road to empowerment as individuals.

Conclusion

Whether or not the health visiting involvement in the slimming group had a long-term, beneficial effect depends largely on whether the women felt that (at the end of the six sessions) their attitudes to food, eating and their own body image had changed, or whether the health visitors had in fact colluded with the myth that to be thin is to be beautiful. The final session suggested that the seeds of a growing awareness of external pressures upon women to conform to a certain body shape had been sown, and that overall the growing self-esteem within the group seemed to override any tensions which had hitherto existed. Unfortunately, due to lack of resources, the group failed to meet again. One rather unexpected outcome, however, was that the educators, the health visitors, became the educated, becoming increasingly aware of the myriad of beliefs, emotions and fears which underlie the food choices any woman makes. The desire for health and the wish to avoid ill health are merely two of the many other factors influencing women's attitude to food.

This work was small scale and qualitative. Nevertheless, as as means of gaining a picture of people's lives, participant observation is a valuable research too. As Reason and Rowan (1981, p. xiv) point out:

Some things which are numerically precise are not true; and some things which are not numerical are true. Orthodox research produces results which are statistically significant but humanly insignificant; in human inquiry it is much better to be deeply interesting than accurately boring.

References

Atwood, M. (1983). *The Edible Woman*. Virago: London.

Berger, J. (1972). *Ways of Seeing*. Penguin: Harmondsworth.

Blaxter, M. and Paterson, E. (1982). *Mothers and Daughters: A Three Generational Study of Health Attitudes and Behaviour*. Heinemann: London.

Charles, N. and Kerr, M. (1988). *Women, Food and Families*. Manchester University Press: Manchester.

Cline, S. (1990). *Just Desserts*. Andre Deutsch: London.

Coward, R. (1984). *Female Desire*. Paladin: London.

Ellman, L. (1988). *Sweet Desserts*. Penguin: Harmondsworth.

Featherstone, M. (1982). The body in consumer culture. *Theory, Culture and Society, 1*, pp. 18–31.

Featherstone, M. (1991). The body in consumer culture, in Featherstone, M., Hepworth, M. and Turner, B. (eds). *The Body*. Sage: London.

Fieldhouse, P. (1986). *Food and Nutrition: Customs and Culture*. Croom Helm: London.

Graham, H. (1984). Surveying through stories, in Bell, C. and Roberts, H. (eds). *Social Researching: Politics, Problems and Practice*. Routledge & Kegan Paul: London.

Hammersley, M. and Atkinson, P. (1983). *Ethnography Principles in Practice*. Tavistock: London.

James, A. (1990). The good, the bad and the delicious: the role of confectionery in British society. *Sociological Review, 38*, 4, 666–87.

Murcott, A. (1983) (ed.). *The Sociology of Food and Eating*. Gower: Aldershot.

Orbach, S. (1978). *Fat is a Feminist Issue*. Hamlyn: London.

Reason, P. and Rowan, J. (1981). *Human Enquiry*. John Wiley: New York.

Shepherd, R. (1992). Diet junkie in a fix. *Mail on Sunday*, 28 June.

Shute, J. (1992). *Life Size*. Secker & Warburg: London.

Wolf, N. (1990). *The Beauty Myth*. Vintage: London.

24 *Healthy living after illness*

Deborah McCaffrey Boyle

Introduction

How a patient and family chose to adapt their lives after the insult of a life-threatening illness is dependent upon numerous variables, and hence is a highly individualised process. This chapter will review major considerations in the evaluation of patient–family adaptation to illness such as, (i) the demands imposed by the illness (i.e. functional loss, self-care requirements, new skill training, treatment continuation); (ii) the assignation of meaning to the illness (i.e. use of self-blame/guilt, perceived or known potential future lethality); and (iii) the coping style of the patient–family unit (i.e. past history and present context, social milieu in which 'living on' transpires, the future's orientation of the family system.) Varied options for healthy living after illness will be shared citing patient scenarios with acute and chronic illness trajectories. Importantly, an outline describing variables to assist with patient–family adaptation 'beyond illness' will provide the reader with an assessment framework to guide intervention planning within individual clinical practice settings.

'Living on'

Adaptation to acute and chronic illness must be considered a multidimensional, highly individualised response with few predictable norms. However, certain parameters influence and may govern how the patient–family unit reacts to the news of disease and illness (i.e. the diagnosis), the proposed amelioration of the disease (i.e. treatment) and post-therapy changes in the patient–family norm (i.e. rehabilitation and the follow-up care requirements). Heightening nursing sensitivity to these assessment parameters encourages the development of care protocols which are tailored to the specific needs of each patient and thereby acknowledges patient diversity and uniqueness, particularly in reference to other patients sharing similar medical diagnoses. It is this hallmark of nursing practice – this customisation of care interventions

– which sets nursing apart from other health care providers, as nurses not only view the uniqueness of each individual patient, but advocate for this individuality in negotiating all spheres of care with every member of the health care team.

Patient adaptation to illness can be described as a continuum. Beginning with baseline function, this norm serves as the foundation for the initial reaction to the acute crisis. Once the shock of insult to well-being absolves somewhat, then some solidification of the acute reaction, some integration of the reality of what occurred in the patient's health status, transpires. Soon after, a choice needs to be made. How does this acute reaction to the alteration in health status the patient demonstrated fit him for the future? Modifications of this early response must be decided upon, as 'living on' beyond the initial insult of illness poses differing agendas for the patient. For example, the patient may ponder, 'Am I still sick? Can I be healthy while still having the illness?' The intensity of the illness may not be the same as earlier on in the illness trajectory, but the illness's insult to the patient's vision of him or herself as a 'healthy person' has left it's mark. Three major areas must be considered which impact patient decision-making regarding options for 'healthy living after illness'.

Consideration of the demands imposed by the illness

Critical to the mastery of a new life's orientation, now influenced by the reality that the person is vulnerable to disease and is imperfect in function, are the demands pertinent to the patient-specific illness. These may include functional loss (i.e. loss of peripheral vision following a stroke), self-care requirements (i.e. meticulous foot care for insulin-dependent diabetics), new skill training (i.e. flushing atrial catheters for ongoing antibiotic administration) and treatment continuation (i.e. hormone replacement therapy following hypophysectomy). Both the nature and the intensity of the demand influence the patient's willingness not only to learn new knowledge but to assimilate it into his or her new life pattern.

Assignation of meaning to the illness

How the patient interprets his or her illness is a critically important variable in determining the direction of 'living on' after disease diagnosis. Assigning value, meaning and purpose to one's interruption in health influences the degree to which one finds resolution or appears to 'remain stuck' in denial, anger or depression about what has occurred. Often characterised by self-blame, illnesses such as tobacco-related malignancies, chronic obstructive pulmonary disease and peripheral vascular compromise are particularly difficult to move beyond once defined.

The diagnosis of an illness with immediate connotations to dying has ramifications which strongly influence one's perception about 'living on', in both quality and quantity. The nature of the illness (i.e. its new demands on the patient and family unit) and the interpretation of the illness (i.e. its likelihood to cause an earlier than expected death), influences the patient's future orientation and related attitudinal and behavioural change potential.

Patient–family coping style

It is the highly personalised nature of how one copes with crisis that makes the patient's illness trajectory a unique one. Numerous variables influence coping behaviours, as witnessed daily by nurses and the health care team. Some of these to be considered include:

1 General coping style of the patient
   - what is the patient's coping norm?
   - What is the patient's anxiety level? how does it influence information reception and retention?
   - to what degree does a worry orientation supersede an action orientation in its relation to stress?
   - is anger a predominant force in coping?
   - how much does the patient want to know about their illness?

2 Health-related coping style
   - what past experiences with disease has the patient had? what was the reaction to this? how are current expectations for recovery influenced by these past experiences?
   - how has the patient coped with past compromise?
   - what is the patient's interest in learning skills of wellness and self-care?

3 Level and nature of family support
   - who is available and willing to render support?
   - what is the developmental stage of the family? what major tasks are they coping with as they evolve as a family?
   - is there other concurrent trauma which is also being addressed by the family?
   - what investment does the family have in promoting recovery and future wellness v. supporting illness behaviours?

Both patient and family variables will modify the direction of illness continuation behaviours or wellness promotion new skill development. Action-oriented patients who maintain hope about their recovery will often enter into partnerships with the health care team to change lifestyles, and seek new options while continuing adjustments to function are implemented. A select subgroup of patients will actively participate in volunteer activities for other patients in an attempt to 'give back' some measure of their positive fortune to those at different points in their illness continuum.

Conclusion

Although exhibiting flexibility in response to life's challenges is a beneficial orientation to becoming healthy after illness, so is a determination to fight rather than succumb to an insult in health status. There is no set recipe to outline to determine how a patient will 'live on' after illness is diagnosed or what might be the best strategy to undertake to ensure a positive outcome. Rather, a highly individualised approach to assessment and intervention-planning optimises the chances for 'healthy living after illness'. Nursing's help during difficult times of transition, such as the phase of re-entry after acute illness, entails giving preparatory guidance and creating an extended care plan that reaches out into the community, with advice that is personally relevant to the patient and practical in nature.

'Living on' in a healthy mode after the initial insult of illness requires both the patient's partnership in attitude and behaviour modification, as well as the nurse's skill and creativity to construct a plan of continued care which is customised to individual patient variables. As many patients and families acknowledge 'things will be different now', the nurse is in a strategic position to help them construct a 'new norm' for their family's functioning. As Brenner and Wrubel (1989) so eloquently states, 'Nurses become experts at coaching a patient through an illness. They take what is foreign and fearful to the patient and make it familiar and thus less frightening.'

References

Brenner, P. and Wrubel, J. (1989). *The Primacy of Caring: Stress and Coping in Health and Illness.* Addison-Wesley: Menlo Park, Cal.

Connelly, C. E. (1987). Self-care and the chronically ill patient. *Nursing Clinics of North America, 22,* 3, 621–9.

Frank-Stromborg, M. (1986). Health promotion behaviors in ambulatory cancer patients: fact or fiction? *Oncology Nursing Forum, 13,* 4, 37–43.

Mishel, M., Padilla, G., Grant, M. and Sorenson, D. (1991). Uncertainty in illness theory: a replication of the mediating effects of mastery and coping. *Nursing Research, 40,* 4, 236–40.

Mullan, F. (1984). Re-entry: the educational needs of the cancer survivor. *Health Education Quarterly, 10* (Special Supplement), 88.

Pollock, S. E. (1986). Human responses to chronic illness: physiologic and psychosocial adaptation. *Nursing Research, 35,* 2, 90–5.

Welch-McCaffrey, D. (1986). To teach or not to teach? Overcoming barriers to patient education in geriatric oncology. *Oncology Nursing Forum, 13,* 4, 25–31.

Welch-McCaffrey, D. and Lyall, J. (1991). Surviving cancer. *Nursing Times, 87,* 32, 26–30.

25 Teaching aids: a study of school nurses' views of their role in HIV/AIDS education

Jane Goodeve

Introduction

The importance of developing effective HIV/AIDS education for young people cannot be over emphasised. Several recent studies have indicated that sexual activity amongst young people (ages 11–19) is common; an estimated 50 per cent of 16 year olds, for example, have had one or more sexual partners (AIDS Newsletter, 1992, p. 7). Sexual contact is the principle mode of transmission of HIV, the AIDS virus. Considering the behaviour patterns amongst this client group, it would seem that the risks of spreading both HIV and other sexually transmitted diseases is a well-warranted concern. Furthermore, the World Health Organisation states that educational programmes should be aimed at children and teenagers before they engage in sexual experimentation (WHO, 1988). Consequently, it is critical that effective strategies for this group are developed.

In the absence of a vaccine against AIDS, it is clear that preventive efforts will depend on effective education (Eisenberg, 1990). However, considerable debate exists as to the nature and content of educational strategies for young people. Furthermore, though a wide range of professionals is willing to acknowledge the urgent need for effective programmes for this age group, few are eager to accept responsibility for their implementation. Without doubt, HIV/AIDS educational programmes for young people raise many sensitive issues.

Health education has been defined as a communication activity aimed at enhancing the well-being and preventing or diminishing ill health in individuals or groups. This may be achieved through favourably influencing the knowledge, beliefs, attitudes and behaviours of those with power, or those of the community at large (Tannahill, 1985). It involves promoting health; a process which enables people to have increased control over and improvement of their health.

The important relationship between schools and health education has been suggested in the literature. Schools have been described as 'health promoting communities'. Images such as this place a substantial amount of responsibility on school nurses. Several researchers and professional organisations have emphasised the important role of school nurses in this regard. Neilsen (1989), for example, describes school nurses as the prime source of information and as facilitators for health promotion and health education in schools for teachers, parents and pupils. Haines (1989) notes that school nurses are situated as a link between health and educational services, in an excellent position to foster and develop health education within the school setting.

In the last few years, recommendations have been made with regard to the role school nurses should play in HIV/AIDS education for young people. The Health Visitors' Association in 1987, for example, stated 'that perhaps the most significant newly emerging health issue is AIDS. Health visitors and school nurses have a critical role to play in primary prevention by supplementing and elaborating upon the information supplied by the mass media campaigns regarding the transmission of the human immunodeficiency virus'. In addition, the United Kingdom Central Council for Nursing Midwifery and Health Visiting (1989) has outlined the important role for nurses, midwives and health visitors in dispelling the myths associated with HIV/AIDS.

Little if any consideration has been given to school nurses' views regarding their potential role in HIV/AIDS education. Few studies have been conducted to explore their feelings about undertaking this role, or their desire and preparedness to do so. It was felt that before these recommendations could fruitfully be put into practice, school nurses need an opportunity to express their views, feeling and concerns about this important topic.

A small research project was designed with these issues in mind. 'Teaching AIDS' was designed to explore and address the concerns of three school nurses with regards to their role in health education and sex education generally, and HIV/AIDS education specifically. Objectives for the study included:

1 To gain insight into how school nurses perceive their role as health educators, with particular reference to the issues surrounding HIV and AIDS, and to identify any problems that school nurses may have in undertaking these roles.
2 To develop three separate HIV/AIDS teaching programmes with school nurses, utilising different methods to teach about HIV/AIDS.
3 To evaluate and compare the effectiveness of the teaching methods in influencing young people's knowledge, attitudes and beliefs about HIV/AIDS.

The remaining discussion will focus on the methods chosen to address the first study objective. Study findings, and relevant issues raised will also be discussed.

Method

The school nurses were drawn from a District Health Centre in West London. Permission was obtained from the school nursing adviser to conduct the study. This particular site was chosen because several HIV/AIDS teaching packages had recently been developed by the local health authority, and the school nurses were eager for the opportunity to try them in practice. A convenience sample was drawn from the school nurses in the health authority.

A semi-structured interview was chosen to explore how the school nurses perceived their role as health educators. An interview schedule was developed to guide question phrasing and recording of responses. The schedule was composed of open and closed questions, thus offsetting the strengths and weaknesses of the two types of questioning. The interview was designed to explore the school nurses' views about health education generally, and more specifically how they perceived their role with regard to sex education and HIV/AIDS education. Questions were designed to assess how prepared school nurses were to take on this role; the instrument was developed with reference to the available literature and in consultation with an AIDS specialist nurse, and a senior lecturer with significant research experience.

Responses were recorded through a process of note taking by the researcher. Upon completion, the interviews were analsyed using a combination of qualitative and quantitative methods. The data was coded to identify persistent words, phrases, themes or concepts. The closed questions were subject to quantitative analysis.

Findings

The school nurses interviewed varied considerably in terms of their age and experience; ranging from 30 to 45 years of age. Initially, the nurses were asked in what ways they felt their role had changed. All three of the nurses felt that their role had changed considerably since they had qualified, with increased surveillance and screening being the areas of greatest change noted by all of them. The significant contribution to be made by health education was mentioned by two of the nurses. School nurse 1 stated 'that the school nurse is the main health educator in schools for both parents, pupils and staff'. All three felt very positive about their role in the future; two of the nurses felt that there was potential for increased specialty in areas such as diabetes and AIDS education.

The nurses were also asked to address their role more specifically as health educators. On a scale of 1 to 10 (with 1 being the most important and 10 being the least important), health education was placed in the top 3 for all the nurses. Topics that they had covered in the past included hygiene (mentioned by 3 of the nurses), smoking (3), reproduction (3), vermin (2), teeth (2), exercise (2), sex (2), drugs and alcohol (2), HIV/AIDS (2), emotional problems (2), family planning (2), foot health, sleep and safety (1). These findings are similar to those of previous studies (HVA, 1987).

Health education was seen as a priority for the nurses in this study. School nurse 2 summed this up nicely, stating that 'health education gives people the knowledge to look after themselves'. This view reflects the WHO (1984) definition of health education as a process which enables people to have increased control over their health.

With regard to sex education, all three of the nurses thought that it was an important part of their role. Reasons for this varied; one of the nurses felt that parents were responsible in an ideal world, but because sex is often seen as a taboo subject this was unfortunately not always the case. Another nurse felt responsible for teaching sex education because 'somebody has to do it; somebody with the knowledge and the ability to teach; somebody to give answers, but also to listen' (school nurse 3).

However, the school nurses' role with regard to HIV/AIDS education seemed to pose some problems. In theory all three of them felt that it was an important part of their role. One of the nurses said, 'if we don't do it who will; it is something that won't go away. Because it is receiving so much attention, there are a lot of misconceptions and fallacies' (school nurse 3). Another summed up the importance of their role, stating 'AIDS is the biggest danger disease in our society at this time' (school nurse 1).

Interestingly, only one of the three nurses interviewed felt prepared to teach HIV/AIDS education. The two others thought that more formal training would be needed before they would be prepared to do so. In discussing HIV/AIDS education in more detail, the nurses agreed on the points to include in an HIV/AIDS teaching session. Two of them said that it would be essential to include modes of transmission of the virus, and also how the virus was not transmitted. Two of the nurses agreed that there are so many myths surrounding HIV and AIDS that knowledge about the disease must be clarified.

The nurses had mixed feelings about who they would include in an HIV/AIDS education session for young people. All three of them felt that they would not separate the children by gender; one said that it would be important to involve parents; two of the nurses suggested it would be important to include teachers, and two would include other health professionals. One of the nurses asserted that it would be important to involve an AIDS specialist nurse in the teaching.

Generally, the nurses were in agreement about how the subject should best be handled. All three felt that small group discussion would be most suitable and that information packs would be very useful. Two of the nurses thought that a question and answer period or an open discussion would be useful for this topic. The nurses had heard of specific AIDS teaching packs but could not remember details. None of the nurses had used a teaching pack in previous sessions.

Issues emerging from the study

Overall, the nurses were very positive about *their* potential role in HIV/AIDS education. However, several areas of concern were consistently expressed throughout the study including the need for preparation in the area of HIV/AIDS, and the need for further collaboration with other health professionals and teachers.

The nurses requested further specialist training in the area of HIV/AIDS. In-service training, videos and television were cited as their preferred information sources. One of the nurses also suggested small group discussion amongst the nurses themselves, stating that 'we need to discuss our views and attitudes about HIV/AIDS if we are to educate the public about this topic' (school nurse 3). Another described what she felt was a serious problem with HIV/AIDS education, namely that 'we need more specialist knowledge on the topic or else we could do damage. Family planning at least has some boundaries. HIV/AIDS doesn't yet' (school nurse 1). These concerns reflect those found in the literature with reference to the lack of statutory training for school nurses (Bagnall, 1989).

It was also felt that further cooperation from the schools would be beneficial. All three of the nurses agreed that school nursing had to become more of a priority, but according to one of them, this is often a problem since children at school are mostly seen as well (school nurse 1). Previous studies have shown that there is often an incongruity between how school nurses perceive themselves and how schools perceive them (Holliday *et al.*, 1984).

The nurses in this study expressed a need for further collaboration with both health and educational professionals. Previous researchers have made similar recommendations (Whitmore *et al.*, 1982; Holliday *et al.*, 1984). It would seem that collaboration is particularly important in an area such as HIV/AIDS where messages to data have been quite unclear. It is imperative that clear and concise messages about HIV/AIDS be delivered if health education initiatives in this area are to be effective. Collaboration of professionals may be one means through which myths about the disease may be dispelled.

However, adequate preparation for HIV/AIDS education and collaboration amongst professionals will only take place if school nurses are supported in undertaking this challenging role. Although several professional organisations have emphasised the important role of school nurses in HIV/AIDS education, at the time of this study few initiatives existed to support the nurses in fulfilling this task.

Of particular interest were the lack of policy initiatives in this area. Shortly after completion of the study (summer, 1991), several significant steps were taken in this regard resulting in the formulation of policy guidelines for HIV/AIDS education in schools. New curriculum requirements were published in December 1991 by the Department of Education and Science, outlining that HIV/AIDS be taught as a compulsory subject to students aged 11–14 years (Department of Education and Science, 1991). Guidelines such as these are an essential step in fostering further collaborative efforts between school nurses and teachers.

Finally, many of the school nurses views about HIV/AIDS education reflect concerns expressed in other circles. Of primary concern is the problem of achieving a balance between the urgent need for HIV/AIDS education for young people and sensitive handling of many of the controversial issues surrounding the virus. Opponents of HIV/AIDS education for young people argue that efforts corrupt rather than inform; topics such as same sex partnership, intravenous drug abuse, and teenage sexual activity expose young minds needlessly to corruption.

The school nurses interviewed, however, felt strongly that HIV/AIDS education for young people is essential. A brief look at other study findings indicate that their views are well supported. A recent study found that most girls aged 11–17 years had become sexually active before they had received contraceptive advice, and that most young people cited friends as the most common source of information about HIV/AIDS (Family Planning Association, 1992).

Such findings suggest that the concerns expressed by school nurse 3 are justified. There are many myths and misconceptions about HIV/AIDS and there is a strong argument for enhancing HIV/AIDS education for young people. Information must be handled sensitively, delivered in a supportive environment and be grounded in sound professional training. This will provide the first step towards ensuring that young people are informed and protected for the future. At the moment, these efforts are our only weapons against the deadly AIDS virus. It is our responsibility that they are used.

Acknowledgements

This study would not have been possible without the support of the school nurses who participated. The researcher also wishes to express special thanks to Dr Alison While and Mrs P. Bagnall for their enthusiastic support throughout the study.

References

AIDS Newsletter (1992), 7, 10–11. Bureau of Hygiene and Tropical Diseases: London.

Bagnall, P. (1989). School nursing: time to face the future. *Health Visitor*, *62*, 7, 224.

Department of Education and Science (1991). *Curriculum Statutory Instrument.* HMSO: London, 15–16.

Eisenberg, L. (1990). Health education and the AIDS epidemic, in Doxiadis, S. *Ethics in Health Education*. John Wiley: London.

Family Planning Association (1992). Cited in AIDS Newsletter (1992), 7, 3.

Haines, M. (1989). School nursing in Norwich Health Authority. *Health Visitor*, *62*, 531–2.

Health Visitors' Association (1987). *Health Visiting and School Nursing Reviewed.* HVA: London.

Holliday, K., Carter, E. and Cardwell, E. (1984). The school nurse as health educator. *Health Vistor*, *57*, 182–3.

Neilsen, M. (1989). The changing role of the school nurse within Worcester and District Health Authority. *Health Visitor*, *62*, 349–50.

Nursing Times (1992). Cited in AIDS Newsletter (1992), 7, 3.

Tannahill, A. (1985). What is health promotion? *Health Education Journal*, *44*, 4.

United Kingdom Central Council for Nursing, Midwifery and Health Visiting. (1989). *Statement on AIDS and HIV infection*. Circular PC/89/02, 6 November.

Whitmore, K. *et al.* (1982). Health services in the primary schools: the nurse's role. *Nursing Times* (8 September), 103–4.

World Health Organisation (1988). *WHO AIDS Series: Guidelines for the Development of a National AIDS Prevention Control Programme*. WHO: Geneva.

World Summit of Ministries of Health on Programmes for AIDS Prevention (1988). 26–28 January. Pergamon Press: Geneva.

26 Occupational health policies for the health service

Sarah E. Adams

This business of health – the National Health Service as an employer

Since the work of Sir William Beveridge, and later Bevan, which culminated in the formation of the National Health Service (NHS), in 1948, there have been many political changes which have affected the way in which our health care system operates. The changes have led to an almost constant revision of policies and programmes within the NHS. A series of reports have been commissioned since 1948, assessing the health care needs of the nation and ways in which these needs can be met.

One such report was the Black Report. The working group for the Black Report completed its review in 1980. In essence, it found that the poorer health experience of the lower occupational health groups applied to all stages of life. 'The Working Group argued that much of the problem lay outside the scope of the NHS. Social and economic factors, such as income, work (or lack of it), environment, education, housing, transport and what are today called "lifestyles" all affect health and favour the better off' (Black *et al.*, 1988). It is not only the NHS that influences the health of our nation, but it has been recognised more recently that it has a leading role to play and the emphasis of the health care provision needs to be changed. Health promotion can be targeted at all social and economic groups and those in work can be considered as a group in themselves. This chapter considers the provision of policies and programmes for promoting the health of those working in the NHS with support evidence from a recent survey.

Historically, the starting point for the NHS has been the services which it provides for its patients in hospitals. Advances in medical and surgical technology allow a demanding few to extend personal life expectancies at an enormous cost to the service provider and to the tax payer. Given the current financial crisis in the National Health Service, both the public system and private insurance agencies have become very interested in the potential for reducing health care costs through the practice of preventive medicine. Cheaper and more effective health delivery systems which place emphasis on prevention rather than cure have been slow to develop, being hampered by lack of funds and commitment to change. However, the publication entitled *The Health of the Nation* states that it will be health problems that we are seeking to avoid. *The Health of the Nation* focuses on health rather than treatment of illness.

The National Health Service is the single largest employer in the United Kingdom, and as such is ideally placed to influence the health of a large proportion of the adult population. Through good employment practices, the provision of occupational health services and health promotion, the NHS has the opportunity to maintain, promote and improve the health of its employees. As an employer, the NHS draws on many who fall into the lower occupational groups, as identified in the Black Report: those who are poorly paid, those who experience work overload or underload; those whose cultural background, language and education place them in the lower occupational group. These employees are often resident locally to their place of work and reflect the very health care needs of the community. At work, the employee can be helped to promote good health through policies and programmes which, when appropriately resourced, can assist people to correct poor health practices. By promoting good health and preventing illness in its own workforce, the NHS has another opportunity to influence further the health of local communities. There is much evidence to show that significant improvements in health can be brought about by raising people's awareness.

Health promotion includes passing on information about how illness is caused and how accident, injury and disease can be avoided. The NHS workplace provides an ideal location for developing this concept, and as an employer there is a further incentive to reduce employment costs and protect the investment that is made in human resources.

Few steps have been taken so far to coordinate the provision of health care for NHS staff. Despite the General Whitley Council agreements, within each Region, District Health Authority and Trust, there are variations in the procedures for staff selection, recruitment and retention. There is no overall standard for the supervision of employee health. Policies and practice for pre-employment health assessment, managing absence and health surveillance of employee groups are conducted in many ways with varying degrees of quality and continuity. Work has recently commenced amongst small groups of dedicated practitioners to audit occupational health practices in the NHS and during 1992 a study was commissioned on this very subject which is being carried out at the Institute of Occupational Health at Birmingham University.

The official government acceptance in 1984 of the Health for All policy, adopted by thirty-two countries within the World Health Organisation (WHO) European, provides a valuable framework for adopting workplace health policies (WHO, 1985a). Of the thirty-eight European Health for All targets, several agree with an existing philosophy fundamental to workplace health: healthy choices (target 13); social support systems (target 14); educational programmes (target 15); health promotion (target 16); and healthy working conditions (target 25).

There can be no better place to start working towards these targets than in the National Health Service itself. Preventive medicine in the workplace is not only a means of improving the health of the workforce but it is a powerful vehicle by which the image of the NHS can be developed. Health promotion in the NHS workplace can reinforce efforts to maintain, promote and improve the health of the community. *The Health of the Nation* documentation states that there will be an initiative to secure better health for staff working in the NHS. Efforts are now being made at national, regional and local level to identify the policies and programmes that exist now and work must be done towards achieving this objective. In considering the value of better health, it is recognised that there is an enormous cost to the employer and to the British economy of avoidable illness in the workforce. This includes working days lost and expensive treatments provided where accident and illness could have been prevented. There is an obvious economic benefit to the NHS if better health can be achieved for those working in it.

To assess the current employee health promotion policies and programmes in the National Health Service, a sample survey was conducted in July 1992 of both health promotion and occupational health departments in the NHS. Occupational health departments were selected as a comparison with the Health Promotion Units because the core ingredient of all occupational health activity is prevention. The common functions of NHS occupational health services include: screening for and offering protection against occupational disease, implementing health and safety programmes, providing periodic health surveillance and health assessments. All these functions share prevention as an underlying principle and provide frequent opportunities for health education and the promotion of good health.

An identical questionnaire was used for both health promotion and occupational health departments but with appropriate headings and terms of reference. For each category, 100 questionnaires were sent out by random selection of the 194 District Health Authorities of the fourteen Regions of England.

The questionnaire was mailed with a covering letter which explained the purpose of the survey:

- to consider the issue of health promotion for National Health Service staff; and
- to demonstrate the current level of health promotion commitment and activity within the National Health Service, in its capacity as employer.

The overall response rate was 63 per cent; health promotion responses amounted to 66 per cent and occupational health slightly less at 60 per cent.

Ninety-nine per cent of the Health Promotion Units were either part of a District Health Authority or Trust – the remaining 1 per cent did not specify, whereas 80 per cent of the occupational health respondents claimed to be part of an authority or trust. Whilst it is more likely that some occupational health services provided by external contractors, it is accepted that the ambiguity of the opening question may have led to unclear responses.

The second part of the first question asked: 'Does your employing Authority or Trust have a policy statement relating to the health and welfare of its employees?' Answer Yes or No. *Table 26.1* shows the responses. From the findings shown in *Table 26.1*, the first observation is that many of the non-responders were apparently unsure of the answer, this being confirmed by most qualifying their response with 'don't know'. For both parties it seems that there is a lack of communication in each employment situation – neither the occupational health nor health promotion respondents knew what statements had been made about employee health, given that the meaning of the question was understood. Whilst some employers may believe they have a commitment to staff health, this may not have been communicated to the levels where policies and programmes are implemented.

Table 26.1 *The response to question 1.2 (percentages)*

Occupational health:	Yes	68
	No	24
	No response	8
	Total	100
Health promotion:	Yes	48
	No	37
	No response	9
	Total	100

Second, amongst the Yes responders there were many supplementary remarks which gave examples of policies such as: smoking, alcohol and health and safety. These examples suggest that some employers have looked at specific aspects of health and welfare but not towards comprehensive 'employee health/welfare' policies. It is after all, a statutory obligation for the employer to have a Health and Safety Policy where there are five or more employees (Health and Safety at Work Act, HMSO, 1974).

Respondents were asked to supply such information as they felt able. Eight separate employing trusts/authorities returned information; the oldest work was dated 25 November 1980 and the most recent were two documents relating to the launch of *The Health of the Nation*, dated 1992. In addition, one trust hospital had made a statement in its trust documentation whereby it makes a public commitment to the health of the staff employed. This was the only example that was furnished ahead of the action packs issued by the Department of Health which suggests the development of such policies.

Further answers in the questionnaire showed a high level of professional interaction between the occupational health and health promotion units. The exchange of information between the two services is covered in *Figure 26.1*. The link between the two functions for the purposes of NHS employee health promotion is shown in *Figure 26.2* in which the two departments shared a common interest in policies and programmes such as smoking, alcohol and Look After Your Heart. *Figure 26.1* shows the variety and frequency of policies found amongst the responders.

On the part of the health promotion units, there was a 99 per cent response in favour of occupational health functions having a role in health promotion activities for staff within the NHS. However, three health promotion units responders made a specific point that their colleagues in occupational health were adopting a 'go-it-alone' approach and considered that team working with occupational health practitioners was difficult. This attitude was not borne out by the respondents in occupational health; 99 per cent of them considered that occupational health has a role to play in health promotion activities. This view is much supported by J. E. Asvall who, as Regional Director for Europe WHO, in March 1990, suggested that 'the time has come to stop seeing health at work as being different from health in general. A broader vision of workplace health policy must be employed that will aspire to the major partners (occupational health practitioners, employers, employees and both government and non-government decision makers) to work closer together.' Whilst the survey referred to here is concerned with the occupational health functions and health promotion units of the NHS, it really is not important who promotes health and safety, only that it is recognised as being important and

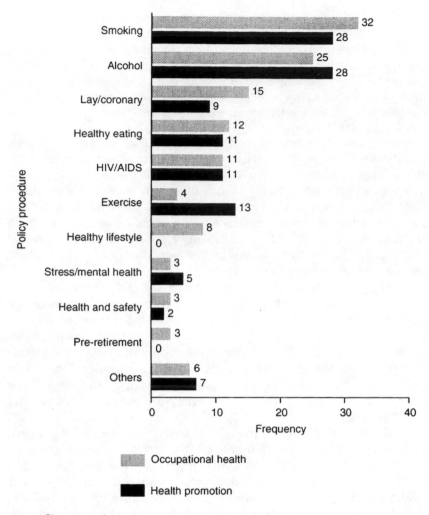

Figure 26.1 *Professional contact relating to health authority policy and/or procedure*

desirable, and that through its commitment, the NHS develops appropriate policies and programmes throughout its purchasing and provider functions.

Finally, the questionnaire considered the issue of resourcing the respective health promotion and occupational health functions. A variety of answers indicated that the health authorities and trusts were still funding both services to staff although several of the occupational health functions indicated that they were conducting 'income generation' work. There is a management expectation for occupational health

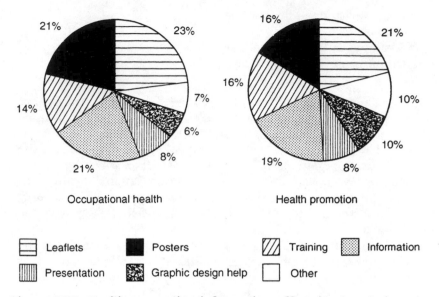

Occupational health   Health promotion

Leaflets   Posters   Training   Information

Presentation   Graphic design help   Other

Figure 26.2 *Health promotion information offered/requested*

services to move towards a state of 'self-sufficiency' and there are real concerns as to whether this may be at the cost of reduced services to NHS employees. Very few respondents indicated that they were used to working in jointly funded projects or had incomes from outside the NHS to conduct activities for NHS employees.

It is suggested that within health care services generally it is difficult to market health promotion for staff successfully and even more difficult to demonstrate the effective use of such intervention. 'Physician, heal thyself' attitudes are still to be found. There is also the traditional misconception that the health carer is able to provide appropriate support for colleagues and staff. Furthermore, the lack of agreed employment policies, involving staff side associations and suitably qualified professionals can detract from the potential for the employer to offer appropriate and acceptable programmes for staff. Despite available publicity and promotion, the role of occupational health functions and health promotion units is often misunderstood and, at worst, not recognised. With this background, it is not surprising that the single largest employer in Britain, the NHS has not developed a wide range of influential and meaningful health promotion programmes.

The survey conducted among occupational health and health promotion services demonstrates that close relationships are already established between these two functions. Common areas of activity include:

- smoking policies and programmes
- alcohol policies
- look after your heart programmes
- nutrition/healthy eating policies
- exercise, and others.

It seems now, more so than ever before, that the opportunity has arisen for health promotion to be taken seriously and for planned strategies to be implemented in the NHS workplace. This view is supported by the European Health for All policy and the Health of the Nation statement of intent to secure better health for those working in the NHS. A workplace health promotion/occupational health programme can make a substantial contribution to controlling not only the physical but also the mental health and social well-being of the NHS employees.

In addition to the effects on mortality and morbidity, there is also the scope to upgrade the physical capabilites in a workplace which is dependent upon a large number of employees conducting physical tasks, such as the manual handling and lifting of patients, for example, the physical benefit of regular exercise, strengthening the back and abdominal muscles, with the improvement of posture. This could reduce the risk of back injury in the individual and could promote, maintain and improve the health of the employee. The survey results demonstrate that a high number of policies are in place already. However, there is a fragmented approach to programmes and procedures enabling a broader preventive approach to be implemented.

WHO has divided work-related disorders into four categories, see *Table 26.2*, which presents a clear picture for the scope of health promotion and preventive practice in the workplace. The classification expands the opportunities for utilising the workplace as a focus for the promotion of health. Occupational health services are already established and, although the policies and programmes are variable, the

Table 26.2 *Categories of work related disease and injury*

Category	Examples
1. Work the direct cause	Lead poisoning injury
2. Work as contributory cause	Coronary heart disease
3. Work as an aggravating factor	Psoriasis, peptic ulcer
4. Work with easy access to potential dangers	Inkeeping: cirrhosis Laboratory: suicide

structure exists to take forward the commitment to secure better health for staff working in the NHS.

A benefit for the National Health Service is that, as an employer, the organisation can be seen to take the lead in developing a national initiative in disease prevention. It can also show other benefits, those of ethical and moral value, professional, legal and economic. To quote Professor Schilling from the *British Journal of Industrial Medicine* in 1989: 'The worksite is the best place for taking action to prevent work related injury and disease. It is an appropriate setting for a broader approach to promotion and prevention'.

To maintain, promote and improve the health of the National Health Service workforce should be our aim. Successful prevention, like good treatment, needs not only a political statement of intent but supporting policies and programmes adequately resourced at the stage of development. On implementation, there needs to be monitoring at all levels and evaluation to enable on-going development of practices that are acceptable and accessible. Through such programmes, individuals can be encouraged through personal and professional contact to take responsibility for their own health. The provision of assessment, information and training is now a feature of many European Community Directives and these are increasingly being reflected in the development and implementation of Regulations under English statute. However, it is suggested here that it is not sufficient to practice to the lowest possible standard set: 'individual workers need to be fully informed and educated so that they can participate in raising the standards of health and safety in the workplace and in making decisions about changing their own lifestyle to improve health' (Schilling, 1989).

There is no doubt that the politics are ripe for health promotion initiatives, the policies and programmes are being developed and work has begun, as shown by the survey. It seems, however, that although the structures are in place and both knowledge and skills are available, the delivery of health promotion to NHS employees is still a long way down the policy-makers' agenda.

Acknowledgements

My thanks to all contributors, in particular to Angela Arnold who gathered the survey information; the staff of Bloomsbury and Islington Health Authority occupational health services for their cooperation and to Pam Duke for her constructive criticism.

References

Asvall, J. E. (1990). Working Paper European Section. WHO: Geneva.
Black, D., Morris, J. N., Smith, C. *et al.* (1988). *Inequalities in Health.* Penguin Books: Harmondsworth.

HMSO (1974). *The Health and Safety at Work Act*. HMSO: Geneva.

Schilling, R. S. F. (1989). Health protection and promotion at work. *British Journal of Industrial Medicine, 46,* 683–8.

World Health Organisation (1985a). *Identification and Control of Work-related Diseases*. Technical Representations Series no. 714. WHO: Geneva.

World Health Organisation (1985b). *Targets for Health for All*. WHO Regional Office for Europe: Copenhagen.

SECTION FIVE

Future directions

Resources for research, education and supportive occupational health services are required. Discussion of how these may be funded and introduced, in Lunney's chapter from the USA and Adams' from the UK (Chapter 26) demonstrate how much could be done and is still needed. However, even greater impetus may come from extra-systal pressure by consumers. Intolerance of paternalistic or impersonal care may be the greatest force for change. Once nurses fully ally themselves with such a consumerist movement the culture of health care will become more healthy!

Skills needed to assert a more client-centred type of care are many. Evidence from the King's study (see Wilson-Barnett and Latter in Chapters 8 and 9) is encouraging in that those nurses who value themselves and their contribution are much more likely to demonstrate open, informative and reflective care. The fact that such nurses were generally more highly educated also gives indications for future investment. More confident and knowledgeable practitioners are needed. Such exemplars of advanced health promotion may be the most powerful models from which to build. Practical guidance and reinforcement of good care could well be created by others working alongside these experts.

This book has hopefully provided some other ideas on how nurses can become better health promoters. One area has yet to be addressed. Personal beliefs and behaviours are powerful factors which may give hidden messages. Valuing one's own health and avoiding risks can provide models for others. Disappointing progress on the reduction of smoking amongst nurses is harmful to the reputation and potential benefit the profession can have. This culture which accepts staff smoking must somehow be better understood. More positive strategies could surely be employed if this is a reaction to stress. Occupational health support for smoking cessation would seem appropriate, for it is clear that wider health promotion may be seriously impeded by such inappropriate habits by staff.

From values to implementation it is obvious that belief systems determine health and health care. Giving time and effort to understand and show respect for others is essential to health promotion. Through identifying participants' preferences and priorities and reflecting these in what is provided, not only could health care become relevant, as the final chapter shows, it could also be more effective. Additional research is required evaluating what is needed to encourage staff change, which specific outcomes are affected and whether consumers become more satisfied if care is more health oriented. Effects on staff morale and relationships should also be systematically monitored. In summary, every component of the health promotion movement needs to be questioned and explored as progress depends on this.

27 Development of a programme of health promotion research

June Lunney

The development of a well-balanced and appropriately targeted programme of research requires continuous analysis of ongoing projects and timely initiatives, to stimulate new or additional research when health care needs change or gaps in scientific knowledge are identified. An analysis of the health promotion research portfolio within the National Center for Nursing Research (NCNR) is presented as an opportunity to reflect on the progress that has been made by nurse investigators, and possible opportunities for the future development of nursing research in this area.

The National Center for Nursing Research was established in 1986 as part of the National Institutes of Health, the research arm of the Public Health Service within the United States Department of Health and Human Services. The extramural division of the NCNR is responsible for administering a programme of government-funded nursing research conducted by scientists at universities, hospitals and research centres throughout the United States.

The budget of the National Center for Nursing Research has increased steadily since its establishment in 1986. *Figure 27.1* provides information about the dollars invested in extramural research by the NCNR and, more specifically, about the proportion of that budget which has been used to fund health promotion research over those seven years.

Since 1986, the NCNR has supported 185 research projects within the Health Promotion/Disease Prevention (HP) Branch of the Division of Extramural Programmes. These projects include the traditional research project (RO1), which is the cornerstone of NCNR's extramural funding, Academic Research Enhancement Awards (AREA), which are budget limited awards targeted to stimulate research in non-research-intensive universities, and First Independent Research Support and Transition (FIRST) Awards, which are also budget-limited awards designed to provide a new investigator with an opportunity to develop as an independent researcher. There is consequently considerable

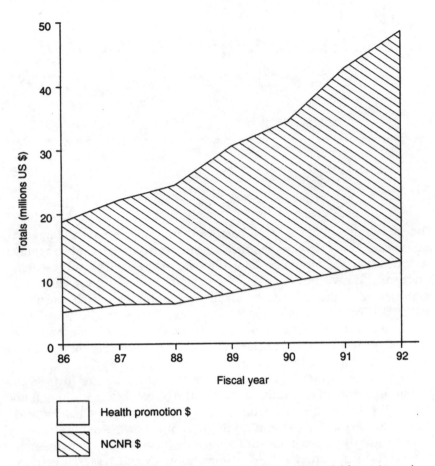

Fiscal year

☐ Health promotion $

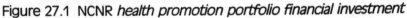 NCNR $

Figure 27.1 NCNR *health promotion portfolio financial investment*

variation in the scope and magnitude of the research goals of the 185 projects. Yet analysed collectively, they provide useful data about the patterns and trends in health promotion research sponsored by NCNR.

The content areas addressed by these studies were analysed using a scheme drawn from a report by Nola Pender and colleagues (1990). These investigators identified six categories of behaviour considered to comprise a health-promoting lifestyle: exercise, healthy nutrition, stress management, building supportive relationships, personal development, and taking personal responsibility for managing health through the appropriate use of health resources. To use this scheme to categorise the content areas of the health promotion portfolio, a seventh category was added concerning the reduction of risk behaviours such as smoking, alcohol use, and unsafe sex practices. Additionally, the category concerning exercise was defined more broadly as balancing activity and rest so that studies of questions related to sleep, respite care, activities of daily living, etc. could be included in this category. In Pender's report, personal development is adult-oriented, concerned with continuing cognitive, emotional and spiritual growth. However, for the purposes of this analysis, the category was broadened to include the notion of normal physiological growth and development for infants and children. Finally, in addition to medical screening behaviours, the category concerned with the appropriate use of health resources includes personal health screening behaviours such as breast self-examination. Studies were coded for multiple content areas when appropriate.

As *Figure 27.2* suggests, more projects have been concerned with the psychosocial aspects of healthy lifestyles, such as managing stress and building supportive relationships, than with other aspects such as nutrition and exercise. Further analysis of the biological versus behavioural orientation of the research also supports this conclusion. The majority (n = 104 or 57 per cent) of the NCNR health promotion projects have had a purely behavioural focus. Only twelve studies have addressed biological questions, and sixty-nine projects were coded as biobehavioural. For this chapter, biobehavioural research is defined very broadly. For example, studies relating behaviours to clinical variables such as sleep, weight gain, and blood pressure were classified as biobehavioural. These data are consistent with a recent NCNR-wide

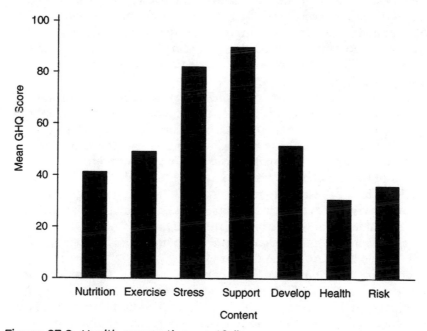

Figure 27.2 *Health promotion portfolio*

portfolio analysis which raised concerns about the strength of the biological base for nursing research (Hinshaw *et al.*, 1991).

The health promotion portfolio was also analysed with respect to the proportion of research that is descriptive in nature compared with that which concerns the testing of a nursing intervention or model of care delivery. One hundred twenty-seven of the 185 projects (69 per cent) represented descriptive research, with nursing interventions tested in 54 projects (29 per cent) and models of nursing care examined in 4 projects (2 per cent). Although descriptive research is critical to knowledge expansion, more intervention research will be needed to develop a sound scientific base for nursing practice.

To explore the nature of the nursing interventions being tested, the fifty-four intervention studies were examined with respect to a second classification scheme drawn from the work of Nola Pender. Both the process (or processes) which characterised the intervention and the desired outcome (or outcomes) were evaluated. Four process categories were identified: direct care, information, skill building, and motivation. Interventions such as activities of the nurse in the neonatal intensive care unit designed to reduce infant stress and promote extrauterine adaptation were classified as 'direct care'. Health education programmes which were concerned only with the dissemination of health information were classified as providing 'information'. Interventions such as those where parents were taught better communication skills with their children or women were shown specific techniques for breast self-examination were classified as 'skill building'. Finally, those interventions designed to encourage healthy behaviours, such as stop-smoking campaigns, were coded as providing 'motivation'. As with the content area, interventions could be coded in multiple categories when appropriate.

Four outcome categories were also identified: change in values, change in knowledge, change in behaviour, and an 'other' category. It was more difficult to operationalise this aspect of the classification scheme. Changes in knowledge and changes in values can be inferred in a behaviour change goal. However, only those projects which specifically articulated an aim to change knowledge or values were classified in this way. Studies were classified as targeted towards behaviour change even if this outcome was only stated as the goal and was not measured as part of the study. Examples of outcome goals which fell into the 'other' category included increased functional status and faster extrauterine adaptation.

As *Figure 27.3* illustrates, one half (n = 27) of the intervention projects contained a skill-building component and sixteen studies (30 per cent) contained a motivation component. This finding is particularly encouraging because behaviour changes were most frequently the target of the intervention (n = 50). Information alone has been

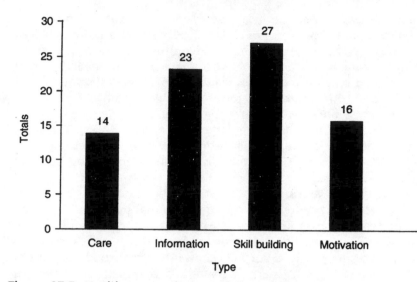

Figure 27.3 *Health promotion portfolio: type of intervention*

consistently demonstrated to be an insufficient change agent with respect to most health behaviours (Damrosch, 1991; D'Eramo-Melkus and Hagan, 1991; Clark and Maclaine, 1992), and it is important to note that nurse researchers are seeking to find effective skill-building and motivational interventions to supplement health education efforts in order to accomplish health behaviour changes.

As one would expect, a large majority (n = 151 or 80 per cent) of health promotion research projects funded by NCNR have been concerned with care provided by nurses in primary care and community health settings. However, this analysis may well under-report the NCNR-funded research which involves health promotion activities for the institutionalised or community-based acute and chronically ill populations. Such projects would more probably be part of the research portfolio of the Acute and Chronic Illness Branch of the extramural programme and not be included in this analysis. It is important that nurses do not overlook opportunities for health promotion in all health care settings.

The distribution of research subjects across the lifespan was also analysed. Four age categories were identified: infants, youths, adults and elders. Projects were coded in multiple categories if, for example, the study subjects included both infants and their mothers, or children and their parents. No attempt was made to code age precisely. If pregnant women were the population of interest, the study was coded as focused on adults, even if adolescents happened to be included, unless the study was specifically directed to the effect of young age on pregnancy. Likewise, older adults were included in the adult category unless the sample was specifically selected on the basis of older age. The distribution shown in *Figure 27.4* suggests that a more balanced portfolio might be created by encouraging future efforts directed at the ageing population. Again, however, there is the possibility that research housed within the Acute and Chronic Illness Portfolio might include a health promotion focus for older adults if they are experiencing acute or chronic health problems.

Of particular interest is the large proportion of NCNR-funded research devoted to issues concerning dyads or families. Seventy projects (38 per cent) addressed issues involving some type of interpersonal relationship. Fifty-seven of these projects were concerned with aspects of parenting. A recent analysis of the entire NCNR perinatal research portfolio also demonstrated that significant attention has been given to parenting, more specifically mother–infant bonding. However, a comparison over time of both the health promotion portfolio and the perinatal portfolio shows that the actual numbers of studies concerned with parenting issues has increased each year, but because of the overall increase in the number of studies, the proportion of resources directed at these issues has declined. Historically, maternal child care was an early focus of nursing health promotion practice. The increasing diversity of health promotion research currently being funded by NCNR mirrors the active role that nursing is taking in the wider area of health promotion research across the entire lifespan.

A final aspect of the health promotion portfolio analysis concerns the gender of the subjects studied. Eighty projects (44 per cent) were concerned primarily with women. This figure is somewhat inflated by

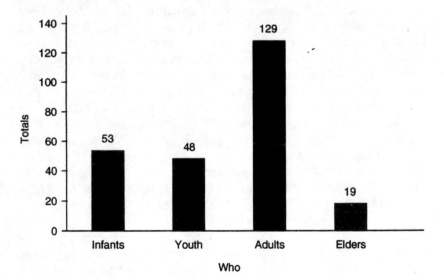

Figure 27.4 *Health promotion portfolio: study subjects*

the decision to code projects which concerned mothers and infants as female-focused (as opposed to parent–infant studies which were coded as representing both sexes). Yet the majority of the eighty projects coded as female (n = 47 or 60 per cent) were concerned with an individual, not a dyad or family. This finding supports the position that nurses have long been concerned with women's health issues, and the NCNR intends to remain actively involved in this area.

The various patterns identified by this analysis of the health promotion research portfolio supported by the National Center for Nursing Research identify both potential strengths and gaps. The increasing diversity of the portfolio and the trend to augment health information with skill building and motivational interventions represent promising signs that nurse scientists are investigating timely questions from the full range of nursing practice. Areas addressed by recent NCNR programme initiatives include the biological basis for nursing practice, the health promotion needs of older children and adolescents, and interventions to foster independence in community-based elders. The ongoing process of thoughtful analysis of the portfolio, together with feedback to nurse researchers and timely initiatives, will contribute to a sound scientific base for nursing practice in health promotion.

References

Clark, J. M. and Maclaine, K. (1992). The effects of smoking in pregnancy: a review of approaches to behaviour change. *Midwifery, 8,* 19–30.

Damrosch, S. (1991). General strategies for motivating people to change their behaviour. *Nursing Clinics of North America, 4,* 833–43.

D'Eramo-Melkus, G. and Hagan, J. A. (1991). Weight reduction interventions for persons with a chronic illness: findings and factors for consideration. *Journal of the American Dietitic Association, 9,* 1093–6.

Hinshaw, A. S., Sigmon, H. D. and Lindsey, A. M. (1991). Interfacting nursing and biologic science. *Journal of Professional Nursing, 7,* 264.

Pender, N. J., Walker, S. N., Frank-Stromborg, M. and Sechrist, K. R. (1990). *Health Promotion in the Workplace: Making a Difference.* Dekalb, Ill.: Northern Illinois University.

28 From sick nursing to health nursing: evolution or revolution?

Jill Macleod Clark

Health care in the UK has reached a watershed and a fundamental shift in emphasis is required in order to ensure that health and nursing continue to be valued. Health care has been manoeuvred into the market place and the principles of cost effectiveness, audit and economies of scale now dominate. The effects of a growth in consumerism and the welcome pressure for enhanced lay participation in health care are also making themselves felt. At the same time, changing patterns of health and illness and demographic shifts are strongly impacting on the demands being made on nursing and health care services.

As a society we have become proficient in prolonging life and preventing death. We have at the same time become more adept at killing ourselves through smoking, stress, and obesity and at acquiring chronic diseases with elusive or non-existent cures. Moreover, the effects of inequality, poverty and disadvantage on health, are increasingly recognisable.

Given this scenario, it is clear that traditional approaches to the education of health care professionals and to the delivery of care are no longer appropriate. In this chapter I will therefore be examining the case for a radical shift in the philosophy which underpins nursing and health care provision.

Nursing research data will be presented to illustrate this need for change and to explore the extent to which any movement along a sick nursing–health nursing continuum has yet occurred. The question is also addressed as to whether such progress is realistically achievable through evolution or whether it requires a revolution of radical proportions.

Much of the research evidence presented takes the form of excerpts from nurse–patient interactions. The methods used in the research in this area commonly involve tape recordings of real life interactions which are then transcribed and subjected to a rigorous interaction analysis process. Examples from these interactions will be used to demonstrate differences in approach between sick nursing and health nursing and the potential enhanced effectiveness of health nursing over sick nursing.

In 1893, Florence Nightingale said: 'Both kinds of nursing are to put us in the best possible conditions for Nature to restore or preserve health – to prevent or to cure disease and injury'. She also wrote: 'A new art and science has been created since and within the last 40 years . . . and the art is that of nursing the sick. We will call the art nursing proper. This is generally practised by women under scientific heads – physicians and surgeons. Nursing proper is therefore to help the patient suffering from disease to live.' At the same time, Nightingale recognised the need for health nursing and her thinking on this provoked the development of the health missioner role – the forerunner of today's health visitor. However, it is important to stress that health nursing was seen as a separate activity and understood by Nightingale totally in the context of health education and prevention of disease – 'to put the constitution of the healthy child or human being in such a state as to have no disease'. It is this perception which still influences the health visitor's role today, with its emphasis on health advice, immunisation and identification of risk factors.

Health education and health promotion in nursing have thus been seen until very recently as the specialist territory or province of the health visitor. When health nursing concepts have been taken on board by other nurses they are interpreted almost exclusively in terms of the activities of health education and health promotion. These activities include health advice, information giving and patient teaching and have simply been bolted on to traditional roles. The reality of nursing practice is that, at best, the activities associated with health education and health promotion have the status of an optional extra. This is elegantly illustrated by the work of Latter and Jones described in Chapters 9 and 10 of this book. It can be argued that by separating out health nursing and sick nursing functions, Nightingale may have seriously hampered the evolution of health nursing.

There is no shortage of rhetoric extolling the need for all nurses to develop their role in promoting health. Indeed the whole of the pre-registration curriculum in the UK (Project 2000) has been revised in acknowledgement of the importance of providing a health focus to nursing education. In spite of this, for the vast majority of nurses, the sick model has remained pervasive.

In sick nursing, care is determined by the diagnosis or problem, care is administered to patients, and expertise and knowledge is owned by nurses and other health professionals. In the same vein, decision-making is dominated by the health professional rather than by the patient or client.

Although attempts have been made to incorporate a health perspective into practice this generally takes the form of 'adding in' activities such as patient teaching and discharge planning. The approach to nursing or the underpinning philosophy of nursing has generally not shifted. Nursing practice remains largely determined by the sick model of nursing rather than by the principles of health nursing.

A health model of nursing encompasses the fact that each individual's need for care is different and that whenever possible, patients and clients should be involved in decisions about and be able to participate in their care. Health nursing focuses on maximising the potential for health and independence. It builds on people's existing knowledge and experience, helps them become more autonomous and empowers them to take responsibility for their own health.

Health nursing is thus the process of promoting health through nursing care. It is vital to emphasise here that it is not what a nurse does that defines sick nursing or health nursing – it is how she does it. The move from sick nursing to health nursing is a philosophical move, not merely a tacking on or a change in the activities of nursing. This is an important point for, by and large, traditional nursing work retains its validity. There remains and will always remain a need to care for the acutely and chronically sick and the dying, and there will always be a requirement to help patients to meet needs they cannot meet themselves. The problem is that the sick nursing approach to providing such care is no longer tenable or appropriate. Sick nursing must evolve into health nursing in order to respond to future health care needs.

In the future, nurses will continue to care for the acutely ill, but their role must also be to prepare patients and relatives for reduced hospital stays and a very rapid transition back into the community. They must help them cope with new demands emanating from high-tech procedures – in effect help them to look after themselves. The increased incidence of chronic disease and the need for rehabilitation will shift the emphasis of nursing care away from caring in the here and now. The focus will move towards giving care which reduces dependency and prepares patients and relatives for the future.

Enhanced life expectancy, the rising number of elderly in the population, and the focus on community care will increase the importance of the nurse's role as a resource and support to lay carers. Growing economic constraints and the market place ethos in health care will place the emphasis on cost effectiveness. Current trends in terms of skill mix mean that professional nurses will find themselves supporting large numbers of less well-qualified care assistants. The growth of consumer awareness and the desire by many to improve their health, remain healthy and be actively involved in their care, constitutes additional but more positive changes.

Taken separately or together, all these changes undermine the value of a sick nursing model. Although well intentioned, sick nursing embodies the principles of prescription, patient passivity and health professional dominance. None of these provides an appropriate basis for meeting future needs. More importantly, sick nursing has no real future because of the type of relationship and interaction it generates between nurses and patients. Such relationships are distinctly 'unhealthy' and are doomed to failure in terms of helping consumers of health to become involved in their care and to maximise their health potential.

However, relationships and interactions will *not* change unless and until the philosophy of sick nursing is rejected in favour of a health nursing philosophy which values the principles of collaboration and partnership.

There are those who believe that evolution has already taken place. It cannot be denied that the importance of health education in nursing has been recognised. Equally the need to offer an individualised approach to care and to encourage patient or client participation is generally accepted. The new nursing education programmes support this insight, but the extent to which all this reflects any degree of true evolution along the sick nursing–health nursing continuum is very questionable. Indeed there is a substantial amount of research evidence to suggest that little evolution has yet occurred. Numerous studies such as those by Elkind (1982), Faulkner and Ward (1983) and Bond *et al.* (1990) have identified deficits in nurses' knowledge about health-related issues including smoking, cancer, HIV and AIDS.

As previously discussed, any evolutionary changes that have occurred are largely restricted to attempts to integrate or add on health education and health promotion activities into nursing practice. This is clearly demonstrated in research by Gott and O'Brien (1990) and the work described in Chapters 9 and 10. The following quotations taken from a study of nurses working in health promotion practice in acute settings (Macleod Clark *et al.*, 1993) illustrates this point:

> Health promotion suggests to me someone who is in need of being taught specific things.

> Health promotion is a system of giving health information to individual patients – it's information giving.

> Health promotion means saying to the patient before they go home about smoking, eating a healthy diet and antistress techniques.

> Health education . . . we try to discourage people from smoking.

These examples are derived from interviews with ward sisters and give some insight into their understanding of the relationship of health promotion to nursing. This understanding is articulated as an adding on of advice, teaching or information giving activities – essentially the sick nursing approach of doing things to patients rather than working in partnership with them.

This suggests that what has happened is that while the what or content of nursing has evolved to some extent, the how or process of nursing and its underlying philosophy has not yet moved. The preoccupation with developing the nurse's health education and health promotion role in terms of activities has perpetuated the status quo of the medical model and sick nursing. Florence Nightingale has proved an accomplice in this through her promulgation of the separateness of sick nursing or nursing proper and health nursing.

In order to bring about change and achieve a philosophical shift, it is essential that nurses focus on the promotion of health at all levels regardless of circumstance, context or degree of morbidity. In other words, the promotion of health needs to become an internalised goal for nurses and indeed all health professionals.

The key to identifying what kind of philosophy underpins nursing practice lies in the relationship between nurse and patient. One of the most potent methods of exploring such relationships is through the observation and analysis of the interactions which take place between individuals (see *Table 28.1*).

Table 28.1 illustrates the fundamental differences between interactions which reflect a health nursing approach and those which would reflect a sick nursing approach. Sick nursing is characterised by patient passivity and dependency, health professional ownership of expertise

Table 28.1 *Characteristics of sick nursing and health nursing interactions*

Sick nursing

Dominating
Generalised
Prescriptive
Reassuring
Directive

Health nursing

Collaborative
Individualised
Negotiated
Supportive
Facilitative

and decision-making and its focuses on care and cure. The relationships between nurse and patient in this model are therefore inevitably characterised by nursing dominance, a generalised approach to care, prescription, reassurance and didactic information or advice giving. Health nursing, on the other hand, is characterised by partnership, patient involvement in care and decision-making, and independence. The relationship between nurse and patient will in turn be collaborative, individualised, negotiated, supportive and facilitative. Health nursing relationships require above all else sophisticated and well-developed communication skills. An acid test, therefore, of the extent to which nursing has evolved along a continuum towards health nursing is through the examination of nurse–patient interactions.

Over the years, nurse researchers have explored and developed techniques for collecting and analysing data in the form of real life nurse–patient interactions. These methods produce high quality audio and video recordings as well as detailed contextual information. Unfortunately, a consistently depressing picture emerges from the analysis of such data. The dominant style of interaction between nurses and patients is that of sick nursing not health nursing (Macleod Clark, 1983; Walton and Macleod Clark, 1986; Macleod Clark, 1987; Cooper, 1991; Kendall, 1991).

In all these studies, interactions were found to be largely nurse dominated, generalised and prescriptive. Our recently completed research on nursing practice in acute settings has also yielded the same picture (Macleod Clark *et al.*, 1993). In the section that follows, examples are given of nurse–patient interactions which illustrate either a sick nursing or health nursing approach.

In the first example of sick nursing given below the nurse is talking to the patient about his medication before he goes home.

N: I'll do a medicine card as well because what we do is write down what each one is for, for you as well and that sometimes helps you to understand what we're giving you.

P: I know what they're for actually, 'cos I've been on the damned things for years.

This represents a classic example of nurse domination and ownership of knowledge and expertise. It also bears no relationship to the patient's own circumstances or needs.

In the next example the scenario is similar, but is dealt with by using a health nursing perspective.

N: How confident are you feeling about taking all your different medicines?

P: Well the wife and me have a list now so it should be OK.

N: Would you like me to run through them again with you?
P: Um, yeah. It would be better if you could do it when she comes in.
N: OK, fine, we'll do that then.

This interaction is clearly focused on the patient's particular needs and is conducted in collaboration and negotiation with him, thus facilitating his involvement.

The two examples that follow share a common theme – that of patients' anxieties about cancer. The way in which these are dealt with, however, differs greatly.

P: I know the lumps have been taken away but it's horrible wondering what they've found.
N: Yes, the tissue is being investigated is the best way to put it.
P: How long will it be before it arrives back?
N: It shouldn't be very long. A few days.
P: You always imagine the worst . . .
N: Well try not to think about it . . . that's the best way. You are in good hands.

Though doubtless well intentioned, the nurse's contribution to the interaction fails to recognise the patient's specific needs and the energy is focused on the time-honoured, sick nursing activity of reassurance.

In the next example a similar situation is handled in a very different way.

P: I'm frightened if I go on the third of February to the hospital and there is something on the scan. I don't know what I'd do – I'm honestly scared.
N: I know, but there's nothing I can say to make that fear go away.
P: No . . . I know it's for my own good and I'd be stupid if I didn't go, wouldn't I?
N: Well, it depends on what you think would be for the best.

This constitutes a useful example of a health nursing approach to a situation. It focuses on the individual's needs, is supportive and facilitates the patient in her decision making.

The next pair of examples are derived from interactions between nurses and patients in the post-operative period.

N: We'll be getting you up out of bed and we'll have to exercise this arm as well.
P: This one?
N: Yes 'cause one of the problems is that it might swell up.

P: Oh, I see.

N: So we'll have to exercise your arm.

Here again an overwhelming picture of nurse dominance is presented. The following interaction provides a stark contrast.

N: . . . you can read that and see what you think. [Puts folder of notes on patient's bed]

P: Am I allowed to read it?

N: Yes, of course you are, it's for you to read.

P: Years ago you would have got your hands chopped off if you'd touched that!

The nurse is talking to the patient about his post-operative care and suggests that he reads his nursing notes. The patient is clearly taken aback – it is not what people have come to expect. However, it does elegantly illustrate health nursing in action – in the collaboration and sharing of responsibility for care and the facilitation of patient involvement.

The examples described above demonstrate the potential value of interaction data in terms of differentiating between sick nursing and health nursing. In particular, they illustrate the fact that in the health nursing examples the nurses are dealing with the main issues and are playing the same role as the nurses in the sick nursing examples. It is not what they do or say that is different but how they do or say it.

This is not in any sense intended to be construed as a criticism of nursing. However, nursing and the health service are faced with an awesome challenge and must be responsive to changing needs and perspective. The medical model and the sick model of nursing will have little value and relevance in the context of future economic and demographic changes and the altered demands for health care. It is also difficult to believe that such models will prove effective in terms of cost and quality in the future. We are rapidly moving into an era which will demand hard-nosed evaluations of nursing inputs. Perhaps one of the reasons that sick nursing has prevailed for so long is that its effectiveness has simply been taken for granted and has not been questioned.

All professionals have a duty and hopefully a desire to evaluate the impact of their interventions. At present in nursing there is a lamentable shortage of outcome studies. This situation has in many ways, I believe, been exacerbated by the prevailing sick nursing culture. The outcomes of sick nursing are elusive and intangible, and often couched in medical model terms such as length of stay and infection rates. Applying and internalising the philosophy of health nursing could open up endless possibilities in terms of identifying health focused outcomes through which to evaluate effectiveness.

In research terms this is the area that we are now focusing on and perhaps where the real academic challenge lies. It is clearly essential to demonstrate a relationship between the process of a nursing intervention and the outcome in terms of patient well-being. In some recent research described in Chapter 22 we have been chipping away at this area. That is, what, if any, is the relationship between how a nurse interacts with a patient or client and the outcome of such interactions? More particularly what difference in outcome is there between using a health nursing and a sick nursing approach?

Much of this outcome research has been undertaken in the field of smoking cessation, which is unsurprising since it provides us with comfortably tight outcome measures which can be validated bio-chemically. Helping someone to stop smoking is very much a two-way process and it will not work in the absence of certain patient–client indicators. Research with coronary care patients has identified some factors which appear to enhance the success of such interventions (Kabat and Wynder, 1987).

One of these indicators is the patient's ability to make an internalised link between smoking and heart disease. What follows are some real life examples of how such internalisation is expressed by coronary patients, who subsequently gave up smoking.

> This heart attack has made me want to give up smoking. Look what cigarettes have done . . . (points to defibrillator marks) . . . I slipped away you know.

> I've had a heart attack and if cigarettes can do that for me, I've got to take this chance now. I could have died that day.

There is nothing surprising about these findings. Indeed it would be strange if there were not a link between such expressions of feelings and subsequent smoking cessation. What must be remembered is that it is necessary for nurses to be working in a health nursing paradigm for such sentiments to be expressed.

Research in relation to the nurse's role in smoking cessation has extended beyond coronary care settings into acute wards and the community (Macleod Clark *et al.*, 1990). The analysis of potential relationships between nursing interventions and smoking cessation again focuses on the nurse's interactive style. Findings show that successful smoking cessation interventions are characterised by a clearly identifiable approach or indicators of the nurses' intervention style (*Table 28.2*). If these indicators seem familiar it is because they are strongly bedded in a health nursing framework. They include individualised assessment and interventions which help the patient to articulate a relationship between smoking and heart disease. In

Table 28.2 *Characteristics of successful approach to smoking cessation*

- Individualised assessment of motivation to stop
- Individualised assessment of health beliefs about smoking
- Internalised acceptance by patient or client of relationship between smoking and morbidity
- Patient or client ownership of decision to quit
- Patient or client ownership of approach to quitting and coping strategies
- Access and use of nursing support and follow up

---

addition there is evidence of collaboration and continued nursing support in the process and ownership of the decision to stop smoking.

Further analysis of the interactions has also revealed a relationship between the communication skills used by the nurses and the subsequent outcomes (ibid.). There is obviously a seminal link between the philosophy which underpins practice and the communication skills which are used to operationalise that philosophy. Mixing a sick nursing model with good communications skills will not result in health nursing – neither will a health nursing model in combination with poor communication skills.

Successful interventions are characterised by specific communication skills, involving open questions, active listening reinforcement and picking up cues. These actively reinforce patient involvement, and most markedly there is a dominance of patient or client talk over nurse talk.

The following extracts serve to illustrate the differences between successful and unsuccessful interventions and they also highlight the relationship between effective interactions and the use of a health nursing perspective and appropriate communication skills. In this next example the nurse is exploring with the patient her feelings about giving up smoking.

N: What particular things worry you about smoking?
P: Mainly cancer.
N: Mmm.
P: I think it's the cancer which has been on my mind.
N: Mmm. So you are worried about cancer?
P: My mother in law, she suffered with it and I was with her 'til the end.
N: Mmm.
P: And she was a terrible smoker. She went through about fifty a day. I wouldn't like to go through that, no.
N: So what do you think you would like to do about smoking?

This intervention is directed at the particular person's needs. It facilitates patient involvement and collaboration and focuses ownership of the issue and decisions about it firmly with the patient. This is achieved through encouraging the patient to explore her concerns about smoking and through the use of active listening and reinforcing skills.

The approach taken in the next example is very different.

N: Do you think your wife would be interested when she hears what you have learned today?
P: I don't think it would honestly bother her 'cause she's got cancer already.
N: Mmm. Yes.
P: But she doesn't relate smoking to cancer anyway so . . .
N: Mmm. What I want you to do is give you a quit smoking contract and to do this contract you really need someone to act as your sponsor so it obviously needs to be quite a good friend who isn't a smoker.

This represents a classic sick nursing approach. It is dominated by the nurse's agenda, it painfully neglects the patient's own circumstances and cues, and is highly prescriptive.

Two further extracts from smoking cessation interventions present very different approaches to helping someone cope with the process of giving up cigarettes.

N: And how keen are you to give up?
P: Well, I know I should give up and I think, I know I would like to, I should be able to give it up.
N: Yes.
P: It's just I think it would be difficult.
N: What do you see as the main problem?
P: The main problems?
N: If you were trying to give up, what would be the main stumbling block?
P: I think it's finding an alternative in something to do other than smoke.

During this intervention the nurse has very much focused on the patient's perspective, gaining his collaboration in the process and facilitating his decisions – a good example of the health nursing approach. This is in stark contrast to the extract which follows:

N: Well, let's start off with a sensible breakfast.
C: I don't actually . . .

N: Go for one of the really high fibre, really filling sort of things.

C: But I don't like them.

In this example the health visitor was offering her solution to the client on how to deal with not having a cigarette first thing in the morning and her concerns about putting on weight. It graphically illustrates the way in which this health visitor's underlying philosophy is reflected in her dominant and directive approach. It is unlikely that a client's smoking behaviour would be influenced by a sick nursing interaction such as this.

The research which generated these examples adds weight to the suggestion that the paradigm which is likely to predict a successful or effective nursing intervention in the area of smoking cessation is that of health nursing. An analysis of the findings from a range of smoking cessation studies which employed either a sick nursing or health nursing approach reveals a similarly compelling picture. For example, studies by Sanders *et al.* (1987) and Sacks *et al.* (1992) both achieved a cessation rate of 5 per cent one year post interventions. These studies were conducted in the community and involved practice nurses, using a stereotyped minimal intervention approach.

A quote from the Sacks paper nicely exemplifies the sick model in practice.

> Each patient had 20 minutes of the nurse's time allocated to them. A personal history was taken and measurements of weight, height, blood pressure and cholesterol were made. Approximately 10 minutes of the appointment was devoted to the anti-smoking intervention which consisted of taking a smoking history, giving information about the risks of lung cancer and heart disease, providing practical advice about giving up smoking, giving leaflets and a follow up appointment date. (ibid., p. 12)

This is a perfect example of the medical model of health education being translated into sick nursing and given that a cessation rate of 5 per cent approximates the spontaneous quit rate, this approach was not successful.

These findings can be compared with the outcome of studies employing a health model for smoking cessation intervention. Such an approach involves individualised assessment and the active participation of the smoker. Research by Macleod Clark *et al.* (1987) and Davies and Evans (1991) resulted in smoking cessation rates one year post intervention of 17 and 25 per cent respectively.

The enhanced effectiveness of a health nursing model is further demonstrated by an examination of the outcome data generated from studies focusing on smoking cessation in coronary care patients. Here we are dealing with a highly motivated group of smokers in whom the spontaneous unsupported cessation rate lies at about 25–30 per cent.

Two studies in which a health nursing model was incorporated (Rowe and Macleod Clark *et al.*, 1993 and Taylor *et al.*, 1990) again achieved a very high validated cessation rate of 70 and 62 per cent respectively one year post intervention. Conversely, studies employing a sick nursing approach such as Fuller Bey (1983) and Hall *et al.* (1983) achieved much lower unvalidated rates with coronary patients of around 30 per cent.

Although, to date, research in this area has been small in scale, the findings are compelling and present a working hypothesis which is well worth following up.

They also represent progress in the pursuit of health-related outcomes through which to measure the impact and effectiveness of nursing interventions. We are just beginning to exploit the potential of developing such outcomes which assess nurses' effectiveness in terms of health increments rather than the absence of ill health indicators. Such health indices include changes in lifestyle and behaviour, adaptation and coping with chronicity, and the facilitation of choice and decision-making in care. They will hopefully be developed and refined for use in future research.

The material presented in this chapter supports the view that the evolutionary journey from sick nursing to health nursing has begun, but that we are not yet very far along the track. It seems that the destination is attainable, as illustrated by the examples of health nursing in practice. However, our experience suggests that such practice to date is the exception rather than the rule.

The question remains about whether and how further progress can be achieved. The process of promoting health will only occur in the context of partnership, empowerment and balance. The key to health nursing therefore lies in a total reappraisal of the relationships and interactions between patients and nurses. This is not simply a case of developing better communication skills.

Health nursing will not be achieved until the philosophy underpinning practice is grounded in the principles of enhancing health. A rejection of sick nursing is required in order that the internalised goals of nursing become linked to the promotion of health. Such a rejection must surely constitute a professional revolution. A social and cultural revolution may also be required, to shift the goals and expectations of the other side of the healthcare coin – the consumers. Once achieved, health nursing could of itself become revolutionary. Radically altering the relationship between nurses and patients would effectively empower the nurse as a professional and the patient as consumer. This in turn would impact on the balance of power within the health care team thus potentially reducing medical dominance and dependence on medical intervention.

In 1893, Florence Nightingale said: 'We are only on the threshold of nursing. In the future, which I shall not see, for I am old, may a better way be opened. May the methods by which every infant, every human being will have the best chance of health – the methods by which every sick person will have the best chance of recovery be learned and practiced.' Ninety-nine years later, her sentiments still hold good – the only difference is that we are now only on the threshold of health nursing.

References

Bond, S., Rhodes, T., Philips, P. and Tierney, A. (1990). Knowledge and attitudes: HIV infection and community nursing staff in Scotland, part 2. *Nursing Times, 86*, 45, 49–51.

Burt, A. and Illingworth, J. *et al.* (1974). Stopping smoking after myocardial infarction. *Lancet, 1*, 304–6.

Cooper, S. (1991). Nurses' assessment skills. Unpublished dissertation. King's College: London.

Davies, J. and Evans, E. (1991). The Newcastle community project, in Adamson, S. and Thomson, A. (eds). *Midwives' Research and Childbirth*. Chapman & Hall: London.

Elkind, A. (1982). Nurses' views about cancer. *Journal of Advanced Nursing, 7*, 43–50.

Faulkner, A. and Ward, L. (1983). Nurses as health educators in relation to smoking. *Nursing Times*, Occasional Paper 79, *15*, 47–8.

Fuller Bey, G. (1983). Anti-smoking counselling: an important part of cardiac rehabilitation. *Canadian Nurse, 79*, 17–20.

Gott, M. and O'Brien, M. (1990). Attitudes and beliefs in health promotion. *Nursing Standard, 5*, 2, 30–2.

Hall, S., Bachman, J. and Henderson, J. (1983). Smoking cessation in patients with cardiopulmonary disease. *Addictive Behaviour, 8*, 33–42.

Kabat, G. C. and Wynder, E. L. (1987). Determinants of quitting smoking. *American Journal of Public Health, 77*, 1301–55.

Kendall, S. A. (1991). An analysis of the health visitor – client interaction: the influence of the health visiting process on client participation. Unpublished Ph.D. research report. King's College: London.

Knudsen, V. (1981). Out-patient educational programmes for rheumatoid arthritis programmes. *Patient Counselling, 2*, 77–82.

Macleod Clark, J. (1983). Nurse patient communication: an analysis of conversations from surgical wards, in Wilson-Barnett, J. (ed.). *Nursing Research – Ten Studies in Patient Care*. John Wiley: Chichester.

Macleod Clark, J. (1987). *Helping Patients and Clients to Stop Smoking. Assessing the Effectiveness of the Nurse's Role*. Research Report no. 19. Health Education Authority: London.

Macleod Clark, J., Kendall, S. and Haverty, S. (1990). Helping people to stop smoking: a study of the nurse's role. *Journal of Advanced Nursing, 15*, 3, 357–63.

Macleod Clark, J., Wilson-Barnett, J., Latter, S. and Maben, J. (1993). Health education and health promotion in nursing: a study of practice in acute areas. Unpublished report. Department of Health: London.

Nightingale, F. (1893). Sick nursing and health nursing, in Seymour, L. (1954). *Selected Writings of Florence Nightingale*. Macmillan: New York.

Rowe, K. and Macleod Clark, J. (1993). The coronary care nurse's role in smoking cessation, in Wilson-Barnett, J. and Macleod Clark, J. (eds). *Health Promotion Research in Nursing*. Macmillan: London, 205–216.

Sacks, G., Anderson, F., Lawless, M. and Thorogood, M. (1992). Smoking behaviour before and after attendance at a health promotion clinic in general practice. *Health Education Journal*, *51*, 1, 11–15.

Sanders, D., Fowler, G. and Main, J. (1987). Randomised controlled trial of anti-smoking advice by nurses in general practice. *British Journal of General Practice*, *39*, 273–6.

Taylor, C. B., Houston-Miller, N., Killen, J. D. and De Busk, R. F. (1990). Smoking cessation after acute myocardial infarction: effects of a nurse-managed intervention. *Annals of Internal Medicine*, *113*, 2, 118–23.

Walton, L. and Macleod Clark, J. (1986). Making contact: communication with stroke patients. *Nursing Times*, *82*, 33, 28–30.

Index